Lactation Management II

Edited by
Kathleen Kendall-Tackett, PhD, IBCLC, FAPA
& Scott Sherwood, BS

All royalties go to the
U.S. Lactation Consultant Association.

Praeclarus Press, LLC

Praeclarus Press, LLC

2504 Sweetgum Lane

Amarillo, Texas 79124 USA

806-367-9950

www.PraeclarusPress.com

DISCLAIMER

The information contained in this publication is advisory only and is not intended to replace sound clinical judgment or individualized patient care. The author disclaims all warranties, whether expressed or implied, including any warranty as the quality, accuracy, safety, or suitability of this information for any particular purpose.

ISBN 978-1-939807-38-0

Cover Design: Ken Tackett

Acquisition & Development: Kathleen Kendall-Tackett & Scott Sherwood

Copy Editing: Chris Tackett

Layout & Design: Nelly Murariu

Operations: Scott Sherwood

Contents

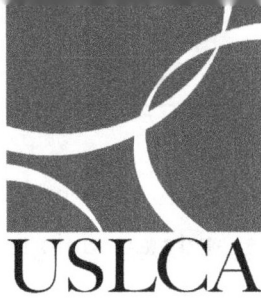

Introduction to Baby Café USA

Lucia Jenkins, RN, IBCLC, RLC[1]

Keywords: Baby Cafe, breastfeeding, United States

Baby Café USA, a nonprofit organization affiliated with Baby Café Charitable Trust of the UK, was established in February 2012 by Lucia Jenkins, RN, IBCLC, RLC, to promote the development of U.S. Baby Cafés, specifically targeting underserved areas with low breastfeeding rates. Baby Cafés are drop-in, free-of-charge breast-feeding support centers that operate by standards and guidelines set by Baby Café USA, jointly with Baby Café UK. Baby Cafés provide crucial support to thousands of breastfeeding mothers around the world and, in addition, gather demographic and statistical data on attending mothers. The UK organization began in 2000, and currently supports more than 120 successful Cafés

1   Lucia@babycafeusa.org, Executive Director, Baby Café USA, Inc., Wake-field, MA, Nonprofit Affiliate of Baby Café Charitable Trust, UK

worldwide, individually funded by a wide range of local community, private, and national grants.

Baby Café USA is the first international affiliate organization to be established outside of the UK and has developed specific U.S. requirements, which include facilitation by an International Board Certified Lactation Consultant (IBCLC). Ms. Jenkins introduced the Baby Café concept to Hallmark Health System (HHS) and Melrose-Wakefield Hospital in 2006. Melrose-Wakefield Hospital opened the first U.S. Baby Café that year, and has opened two additional Women, Infants, and Children (WIC)-based Cafés, all of which HHS continues to fund. Baby Cafés are baby friendly, meet at least once a week, are accessible by public transportation, and offer peer-support counseling, as well as professional-level lactation care. Baby Cafés fulfill Step 10 of Baby-Friendly Hospital Initiative requirements, and are currently open in Massachusetts, Texas, Florida, Minnesota, Alabama, Michigan, Pennsylvania, South Carolina, North Dakota, and New York, with more in the development process.

In addition to tracking exclusivity rates of mothers at Café meetings, Ms. Jenkins has developed statistical gathering tools and a call-back survey to track duration and other factors influencing a mother's breastfeeding experience. This data is valuable to evaluate each Café's impact on community breastfeeding rates. Four years of data from the HHS Cafés are in the final stages of editing and will be submitted for publication in the next few months. Baby Café USA will continue to collect and evaluate all data from U.S. Cafés using standardized statistical gathering tools.

The preliminary results from HHS Cafés demonstrate, for example, that the café model positively impacts the duration goals mothers have set for themselves prenatally: approximately 82% reach their goals, 74% of café moms increase their duration goals, and 71% reach the American Academy of Pediatrics (AAP) goals of breastfeeding for 1 year.

For more information on finding a Baby Café or information on opening a Baby Café in your community, please visit www.babycafeusa.org.

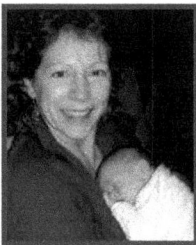

Lucia Jenkins, RN, IBCLC, RLC, is an IBCLC with 19 years of experience, and is the originator and executive director of Baby Café USA. She is a staff IBCLC at Melrose-Wakefield Hospital, has a private lactation practice, and is a board member of the Massachusetts Breastfeeding Coalition. She is the principal facilitator of the first USA Baby Café, and the first WIC Baby Café, both funded by HHS. Lucia has lectured at various conferences and state coalitions, including Massachusetts Department of Public Health (DPH), International Lactation Consultant Association (ILCA) 2009, and United States Breastfeeding Committee (USBC) 2012 about Baby Cafés and the process of starting them.

USLCA

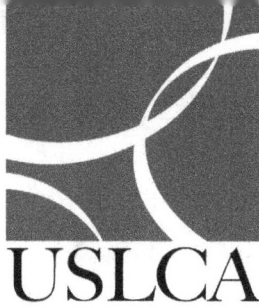

El Paso Baby Café: Peer Support for Lactation Care, Mothers, and Babies

Lizabeth J. Berkeley, MPH, IBCLC, RLC[1]

Wrennah Gabbert, PhD, RN, CPNP, FNP-BC

Josefina Lujan, PhD, RN

Jennifer Whitaker-Ware, MSN, RN

Keywords: Baby Café, peer support, breastfeeding

The use of peer support as a tool to increase breastfeeding exclusivity and duration can be facilitated by innovative community strategies. This is especially important in a binational environment where health care clients are served by providers on both sides of the U.S.-Mexico border. A successful adoption of the Baby Café model of peer-to-peer breastfeeding support, developed in the UK, has been carried out by the El Paso Baby Café and its sister Baby Cafés in Ciudad Juárez and Northern Chihuahua, Mexico.

1   Lizabeth.Berkeley@ttuhsc.edu, Gayle Greve Hunt School of Nursing, Texas Tech University

Peer support for breastfeeding mothers has proven to be an important intervention to increase breastfeeding exclusivity and total duration. This has been particularly exciting for lactation professionals who have been providing care for many years to mothers and babies, and who have struggled to improve support for breastfeeding. A plethora of research on this topic can be found through the Cochrane Collaboration website (Dyson, McCormick, & Renfrew, 2008). When paired with health education, peer support is one of few interventions now universally accepted to improve a mothers' probability of any measure of success.

Recently, there has been an increased focus on supportive interventions by both the *Surgeon General's Call to Action to Support Breastfeeding* (Benjamin, 2011) and the Centers for Disease Control and Prevention's (CDC, 2009), *Guide to Breastfeeding Interventions.* In this vein, now the Affordable Care Act includes mandates for health plans to cover breastfeeding support, supplies, and counseling (U.S. Health and Human Services, Health Resources and Services Administration [USHHS, HRSA], 2011). Simultaneously, breastfeeding is being explored as a concrete, cost-effective intervention to decrease the risk of chronic disease later in life (e.g., obesity), and ultimately to lower economic costs for countries and society at large. National and worldwide public-health institutions are emphasizing peer support of the breastfeeding dyad as a major evidence-based, cost-effective, and positive intervention providing excellent short- and long-range outcomes (Benjamin, 2011; World Health Organization [WHO] Global Strategy, 2003). The U.S. Preventive Services Task Force (USPSTF, 2008) also highlights peer support as one of only four interventions recommended to reliably promote and support breastfeeding. Similarly, the UNICEF Baby-Friendly Hospital Initiative has been recommending the establishment of "breastfeeding support groups and referring mothers to them" for more than 25 years (UNICEF, 1991).

Research has consistently demonstrated the importance of personal connections between women (or lack of connections), and the positive or negative correlation with successful breastfeeding (Jolly et al., 2012; Kaunonen, Hannula, & Tarkka, 2012; Kruske, Schmied, & Cook, 2007; Meier, Furman, & Degenhardt, 2007). Lactation care providers "in the trenches" are not surprised by the increased interest and focus on peer support. Its emergence as both a positive intervention to support breastfeeding, and a pathway for women to connect with other women, makes sense.

The Baby Café Model

Confirmation that peer support is an effective intervention has led to lactation care providers experimenting with varieties of "support" to find the best approach. The Baby Café center model, originating in England (www. thebabycafe.org), is an intervention that offers a unique approach to peer-to-peer support. This model provides free breastfeeding help and support from both health care professionals and other mothers in a nonclinical setting. These "drop-in" centers strive to provide a friendly, welcoming, café-style environment—snacks included—to mothers of all ages and from all socioeconomic sectors of the community (see Figure 1).

Origins of the Baby Café

The first Baby Café was opened in London, England in the year 2000. Currently, there are more than 120.

Figure 1. El Paso Baby Cafe Grand Opening Invitation Flyer

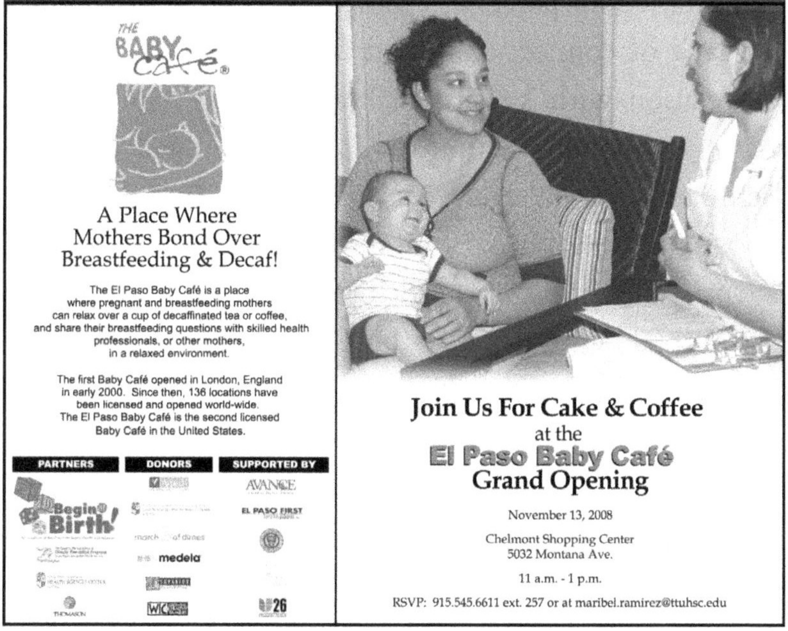

Baby Cafés in the world, and here in the U.S., the pace of openings is accelerating. The first Baby Café in the U.S. opened in 2006 in Melrose, Massachusetts, and the second opened in El Paso, Texas in 2008. Here in El Paso, the model has been implemented on both sides of the

U.S.-Mexico border, in both El Paso, Texas and adjacently in Ciudad Juárez, Mexico. As of this writing, early 2013, there are 17 Baby Cafés in the U.S.

Objectives of the Baby Café

The specific objectives of the Baby Café Project (as set out by the Baby Café UK) are the following:

1. To promote the physical and psychological health of mothers and children through education and training regarding breastfeeding.

2. To advance the general public's knowledge of the health benefits, immediate and long-term, of breastfeeding.

3. To continue education among volunteers supporting breastfeeding mothers.

The Baby Café model works well in both freestanding venues and shared space. Securing donated space has helped many Baby Cafés ensure their long-term viability even when funding sources were exhausted. Hospitals and other institutions whose clients benefit directly from the availability of a Baby Café, and the support service it provides, have shown willingness to provide both space, and a few hours of salary for the lead facilitators.

The United States-Mexico Borderland and the El Paso Baby Café

El Paso, Texas is a large city of roughly three quarters of a million residents that borders Ciudad Juárez, Mexico, the population of which is at least 2 million. The population of El Paso is 80% Hispanic, predominantly young, with a higher fertility rate than the rest of Texas, and a relatively low high school graduation rate (see El Paso County

---

Box 1. Steps We Took to Create Our Baby Café

1. Developed an advisory committee.

2. Created a budget, identified and secured funding.

3. Applied to Baby Café UK for licensing.

4. Identified a venue and lead facilitators.

5. Recruited and trained volunteers and peer counselors.

6. Designed and implemented a publicity campaign aimed at healthcare professionals and the public.

7. Created a documentation system using Baby Café intake forms and tally sheets.

8. Implemented a system for outcome evaluation by Baby Café and funders.

The Baby Café Charitable Trust has recently established a USA affiliate through which all U.S. Baby Cafés are licensed. Baby Café USA (www.babycafeusa.org) provides detailed help and assistance for anyone interested in starting a Baby Café in their community.

Auditor, Budget Book, 2006). Many young mothers arrive at the county hospital with little prenatal education, report low socioeconomic status, and are ambivalent about breastfeeding. These demographics mirror the profile of those mothers most at risk for discontinuing breastfeeding early.

As of this writing, there are only 11 practicing International Board Certified Lactation Consultants caring for mothers and babies between El Paso, Texas; Ciudad Juárez, Mexico; and Las Cruces, New Mexico. Only 3 of those are working outside of a hospital setting. Two are working for the Women, Infants, and Children (WIC) program, and 1 is running the El Paso Baby Café. This deficit of lactation providers was even more acute when the El Paso Baby Café was established.

The establishment of a Baby Café in El Paso in 2008 provided an opportunity to promote and support breastfeeding by addressing two enormous deficits simultaneously: (a) access to lactation consultation, and (b) access to breastfeeding peers. The Baby Café model has been found to be cost-effective, and has raised awareness and respect for breastfeeding in a community where, previously, breastfeeding was rarely seen in public. The creation of Baby Café sites has also provided tremendous momentum and opportunity for specialty training for students in various health care fields (nursing, medicine, nutrition, speech pathology, and pharmacy). It has generated dozens of new peer counselors, and several new board certified lactation consultants. In our immediate region on both sides of the U.S.-Mexico border, there are now seven Baby Cafés.

The El Paso Baby Café (rebranded in 2012 as the Texas Tech University Health Sciences Center [TTUHSC] Gayle Greve Hunt School of Nursing Baby Café) is licensed under the umbrella organization of the Baby Café Charitable Trust UK. One bilingual lactation consultant, and at least one bilingual volunteer, are always available with services offered 4 days a week, 2.0-2.5 hours each session. The lactation consultant facilitates each session and deals with specific lactation problems that a mother might be experiencing (in conjunction with her primary health care practitioner). The volunteers, critical to success, are responsible to make certain client documentation is completed, to ensure interaction with the lactation consultant where needed, to facilitate conversation between mothers, and to help with setup and cleanup.

Contact and communication is maintained with all of the medical/health care institutions in the area through the periodic distribution of Baby Café promotional materials, personal contact, and media exposure. Most maternity care providers (pediatricians, obstetricians, and midwives) have reported becoming familiar with the service either through direct contact, or through media exposure. Over the first 4 years, there have been approximately 6,000 visits by adults to the Baby Café: 1,017 mother/baby couplets visited the El Paso Baby Café from July 2010 to June 2011.

Participation of Community

During the planning stage of the El Paso Baby Café, collaborative community meetings were held in an effort to involve key community leaders and health care institutions, and to inform health care providers of the free service the El Paso Baby Café would provide. The El Paso Baby Café center has received support in the forms of verbal and written endorsements, grants, donations, and in-kind contributions. Organizations that have supported and contributed to the Baby Café in El Paso over the past 4 years include the following: the Paso del Norte Health Foundation; Texas Department of State Health Services: Nutrition, Physical Activity and Obesity Prevention Program; the March of Dimes; TTUHSC Gayle Greve Hunt School of Nursing; University Medical Center of El Paso; City of El Paso WIC; and *Clinica Familiar La Fe WIC*. In addition, the TTUHSC Foundation created a web portal, making tax deductible online donations from individuals possible. Significantly, the El Paso Baby Café received international recognition for its social marketing efforts when it was commended for "Innovative Promotion of the Baby Café" in 2010 by the Baby Café Charitable Trust UK.

> **Box 2. Potential Sources of Funding**
>
> Some potential sources of funding to open and sustain a Baby Café are March of Dimes, your local community foundation, service clubs, women's health funds, WIC, your state health department, fundraisers, donations from healthcare professionals and institutions, and in-kind contributions.

Evaluation Survey Data Results

To assess effectiveness, an informal survey was created and distributed to mothers who had attended the El Paso Baby Café from October 2008 to June 2010. Participants were sent questionnaires in both English and Spanish. There were 450 surveys mailed with 121 (26.9%) returned and included in the data analysis. Major themes and categories were identified in response to the following questions:

> » Have you received information/support from a lactation consultant or breastfeeding peer counselor? There were 85.2% (103) who responded "Yes."

> » Are you aware that mothers are here to help other mothers? There were 86% (104) who responded "Yes."

> » Have you received information/support from another mother at the Baby Café? There were 53.7% (65) who responded "Yes."

> » Did the El Paso Baby Café help you? There were 92% (112) who responded "Yes."

International Expansion Across the Border

One major positive outcome of this program is the rapid growth in the number of visits to the existing Baby Café in El Paso. In addition, expansion into neighboring Ciudad Juárez and Chihuahua, Mexico has organically grown out of a newly identified market. After the first 3 years of operation in El Paso, Texas, local lactation consultants (most of whom were associated with the Baby Café in one way or another) identified the need for Mexican mothers to access breastfeeding support across the border from El Paso in Ciudad Juárez, Mexico. As a result, in 2011, the first licensed Baby Café in Latin America was opened in Mexico (Baby Café Ciudad Juárez—*Instituto Mexicano del Seguro Social* [IMSS]) under the mentorship of the Gayle Greve Hunt School of Nursing Baby Café. The mentoring is accomplished by the use of technology (Skype, email, cell phone) because of the serious security and travel concerns.

Soon afterward, in late 2011, the second Baby Café in Latin America opened, also in Ciudad Juárez. The Baby Café Ciudad Juárez—*Federacion Mexicana de Asociaciones Privadas* (FEMAP) is in a community-based maternity hospital, Hospital de la Familia. A third Baby Café opened in Chihuahua City, the capital of the State of Chihuahua, in the summer of 2012. This third Baby Café, facilitated by a coalition of Nursing School and Medical School faculty in the State of Chihuahua, was initiated by a mother and grandmother who attended the Baby Café in El Paso for breastfeeding help.

Challenges and Recommendations for the Future

The Baby Café's availability to all community members (free-of-charge) makes services accessible to the financially vulnerable. Therefore, it is necessary when contemplating and planning the development of a Baby Café project to continually and actively seek out all feasible avenues for financial support and funding, including foundation grants, institutional support, and private and in-kind donations.

The greatest difficulty the El Paso Baby Café has encountered is in maintaining a sustainable location. The El Paso Baby Café was originally located in a rented space paid for by grant funding. Maintaining the level of funding necessary to sustain this proved to be a tremendous burden on the staff. The provision of donated space provided by the TTUHSC Gayle Greeve Hunt School of Nursing alleviated this problem and has created a secure and accessible venue.

Summary

A Baby Café can be successfully replicated and adapted as a community-based approach to providing effective support for breastfeeding mothers and babies. A tremendous side benefit is the establishment of relationships fostered between clinicians, lactation specialists, clients, volunteers, and concerned community members. The relationships that have been established between the El Paso Baby Café and the community at large, and a growing integration of students in various health care fields into the work of the Baby Café, has been beneficial to overall mother-baby health care environment in El Paso and Northern Mexico. Perhaps the most significant outcome is the mother-to-mother peer relationships that have been created, and have continued beyond the walls of the Baby Café. The mothers and families supporting each other through early childhood and beyond are making strides toward the goal of seeing breastfeeding as the normal way to feed a baby. The Baby Café can provide a pathway for women all over the world to help and support each other to successfully breastfeed.

References

Benjamin, R. M. (2011). *The Surgeon General's Call to Action to Support Breastfeeding.* Retrieved from http://www.surgeongeneral.gov/library/calls/breastfeeding/index.html

Centers for Disease Control and Prevention. (2009). *The CDC guide to breastfeeding interventions.* Retrieved from http://www.cdc.gov/breastfeeding/resources/guide.htm

Dyson, L., McCormick, F. M., & Renfrew, M. J. (2008). *Cochrane summaries: Interventions for encouraging women to start breastfeeding.* Retrieved from http://summaries.cochrane.org/CD001688/interventions-for-encouraging-women-to-start-breastfeeding

El Paso County Auditor, Budget Book. (2006).

Jolly, K., Ingram, L., Khan, K. S., Deeks, J. J., Freemantle, N., & MacArthur, C. (2012). Systematic review of peer support for breastfeeding continuation: Metaregression analysis of the effect of setting, intensity, and timing. *British Medical Journal, 25*(344), d8287. http://dx.doi/10.1136/bmj.d8287

Kaunonen, M., Hannula, L., & Tarkka, M. T. (2012). A systematic review of peer support interventions for breastfeeding. *Journal of Clinical Nursing, 21*(13–14), 1943–1954. http://dx.doi.org/10.1111/j.1365-2702.2012.04071.x

Kruske, S., Schmied, V., & Cook, M. (2007).The "earlybird" gets the breast milk: Findings from an evaluation of combined professional and peer support groups to improve breastfeeding duration in the first eight weeks after birth. *Maternal Child Nutrition, 3*(2), 108–119.

Meier, P. P., Furman, L. M., & Degenhardt, M. (2007) Increased lactation risk for late preterm infants and mothers: Evidence and management strategies to protect breastfeeding. *Journal of Midwifery Women's Health, 52*(6), 579–587.

UNICEF. (1991). *The Baby-Friendly Hospital Initiative.* Retrieved from http://www.unicef.org/programme/breastfeeding/baby.htm

U.S. Health and Human Services, Health Resources and Services Administration. (2011). *Women's preventative services: Required health plan coverage guidelines.* Retrieved from http://www.hrsa.gov/womensguidelines/

U.S. Preventive Services Task Force. (2008). *Primary care interventions to promote breastfeeding: Summary of recommendations.* Retrieved from http://www.uspreventiveservicestaskforce.org/uspstf/ uspsbrfd.htm#summary

World Health Organization. (2003). *Global strategy for infant and young child feeding.* Retrieved from http://www.who.int/ maternal child_adolescent/topics/child/nutrition/global/en

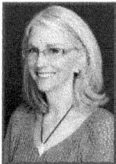

Lizabeth J. Berkeley, MPH, IBCLC, RLC is a faculty associate, Texas Tech University Health Sciences Center, Gayle Greve Hunt School of Nursing in El Paso, Texas, and the director of the El Paso Baby Café.

Wrennah L. Gabbert, PhD, RN, CPNP, FNP-BC is the senior associate dean, Texas Tech University Health Sciences Center, Gayle Greve Hunt School of Nursing in El Paso, Texas. Dr. Gabbert's research focus is on curriculum design for adult learners in a variety of learning formats; her practice focus is on access and delivery of primary health care in under-served and uninsured rural populations.

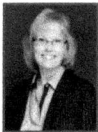

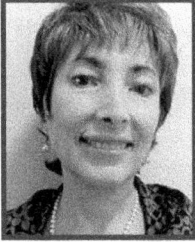

Josefina Lujan, PhD, RN, is an associate professor and associate dean at the Texas Tech University Health Sciences Center, Gayle Greve Hunt School of Nursing in El Paso, Texas. Dr. Lujan's research focus is in U.S.-Mexico border health concerns, Hispanic health disparities, and promotion of diversity in the nursing workforce. She is a life-long resident of the Texas-Mexico border community of El Paso, Texas, where she has practiced as a RN and nurse educator for 33 years.

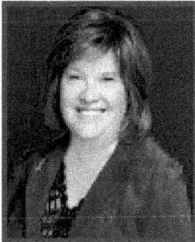

Jennifer Whitaker-Ware, MSN, RN, is an assistant professor of nursing at Gayle Greve Hunt School of Nursing at Texas Tech University Health Sciences Center in El Paso, Texas. She teaches in the Traditional Undergraduate and Second Degree BSN programs.

Resources for Supporting Breastfeeding in Child Care Centers

The Louisiana Breastfeeding Coalition, Our Lady of the Lake Children's Hospital, Volunteers of America/Partnerships in Child Care, and several local breastfeeding coalitions have developed a *Breastfeeding-Friendly Child Care Initiative* to encourage and improve support for breastfeeding in Louisiana child care centers. This toolkit is designed to help Lactation Consultants educate child care providers on best practices for supporting breastfeeding and handling breast milk.

Source: USBC

New Report Available From the Indian Health Service: Indian Health Diabetes Best Practice: Breastfeeding Support

The Indian Health Diabetes Best Practice: Breastfeeding Support report describes clinical tools and technical resources to effectively support breastfeeding. The intent of this report, from the IHS Division of Diabetes Treatment and Prevention, is to assist families in childbearing age that are at risk for type 1 and type 2 diabetes.

Source: USBC

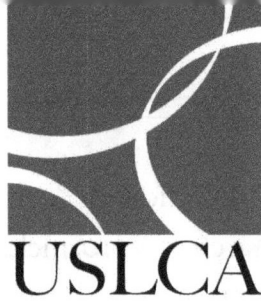

A Time and Place to Pump:

What Lactation Consultants Need to Know about the New Federal Protections for Employed Breastfeeding Mothers

Kori Martin, JD[1]

Keywords: breastfeeding, employment, legal rights

A majority of women in the U.S. return to full-time work during the year after childbirth. According to the Bureau of Labor Statistics, in 2008, 56.4% of women with infants under one year of age participated in the workforce. As breastfeeding clinicians, whether in the hospital or out, IBCLC or WIC Peer Counselor, a vital part of our job in supporting nursing mothers involves helping those who plan to return to the workforce prepare for this future role of balancing breastfeeding with employment.

Now, thanks to a new federal law guaranteeing certain employed mothers access to a time and place to pump while at work, our job just got a little easier.

---

1   Legal Professional Liaison for LLL of Texas, korimartintx@gmail.com

The Patient Protection and Affordable Care Act, which took effect March 23, 2010, includes a provision that amends the Fair Labor Standards Act ["FLSA"] to provide a new federal baseline protection for mothers needing to express milk at work. The text of this law can be found at: http://www.usbreastfeeding.org/Portals/0/Workplace/HR3590-Sec4207-NursingMothers.pdf[2]

What this Law Does

» It requires that employers provide time for their employees to express milk. Specifically, employers must provide "reasonable break time for an employee to express breast milk for her nursing child for 1 year after the child's birth each time such employee has need to express the milk" (FLSA §7(r)(1)(A)).

» It requires that breastfeeding employees have access to a place to express milk. The location must be "a place, other than a bathroom, that is shielded from view and free from intrusion from coworkers and the public, which may be used by an employee to express breast milk." (FLSA §7(r)(1)(B)).

» This provision provides a minimum baseline of coverage. It does not pre-empt any state laws that provide broader protections to working moms

---

2 §4207, Reasonable Break Time for Nursing Mothers, which amends §7(r) of the Fair Labor Standards Act.

(FLSA §7(r)(4)). A listing of state breastfeeding laws can be found at http://www.ncsl.org/default. aspx?tabid=14389

What this Law Does Not Do

» This law does not protect workers who are exempt from the protections of the FLSA's overtime provisions. A mother can find out whether she is an "exempt" or "non-exempt" worker by checking her pay stub or contacting her company's human resources representative ("Request for information," 2010).

» Not all employers are subject to this requirement. Employers with fewer than 50 employees may be able to obtain an exemption if compliance would present an undue hardship (FLSA §7(r)(3)).

» There is no requirement that time used to express milk be paid break time. However, when other employees are already provided with compensated breaks, the law does require that mothers who use their break time to express milk be compensated in the same way as other employees' breaks ("Fact sheet #73," 2010).

» This law does not prescribe requirements as to the frequency or duration of pumping breaks, but instead looks to what is "reasonable" in a given situation. "The frequency of breaks needed to express milk as well as the duration of each break will likely vary" ("Fact sheet #73," 2010), but the WHD "expects that nursing mothers typically will need breaks to express milk two to three times during an 8-hour shift" ("Request for information," 2010).

In developing a plan for break-time pumping, the Department of Labor's Wages and Hours Division ["WHD"], which has been charged with interpretation and enforcement of this provision, suggests that employers and employees work together to "develop shared expectations and an understanding of what will constitute 'a reasonable break time,' and how to incorporate the breaks into the work period." If a mother feels that she has not been afforded the proper time or place for milk expression as guaranteed under the FLSA, she can follow instructions for filing a complaint on the WHD website: http://www.dol.gov/wecanhelp/ howtofilecomplaint.htm

Helpful Resources

http://www.dol.gov/ATimeandPlacetoPump:WhatLactation-ConsultantsNeedtoKnowabouttheNewFederalProtections-forEmployedBreastfeedingMotherswhd/nursingmothers/

http://www.ncsl.org/default.aspx?tabid=14389

http://www.usbreastfeeding.org/Workplace/Workplace-Support/FAQsBreakTimeforNursingMothers/tabid/188/Default.aspx

References

Bureau of Labor Statistics. (2009, May). *Labor force participation of mothers with infants in 2008.* TED: The editor's desk. http://www. bls.gov/opub/ted/2009/may/wk4/art04.htm

Patient Protection and Affordable Care Act, Pub. L. No. 111-148, §4207 (2010). Available at http://www.usbreastfeeding.org/ Portals/0/Workplace/HR3590-Sec4207-Nursing-Mothers.pdf

U.S. Department of Labor: *Wages and Hours Division. Request for information on break time for nursing mothers, 75 Federal Register 80073-80079* (Dec. 21, 2010). http://webapps.dol.gov/ FederalRegister/HtmlDisplay.aspx?DocId=24540&Month=12&Y ear=200

U.S. Department of Labor: Wages and Hours Division. *Fact Sheet #73: Break Time for Nursing Mothers under the FLSA* (revised 2010, December). http://www.dol.gov/whd/regs/compliance/ whdfs73.htm

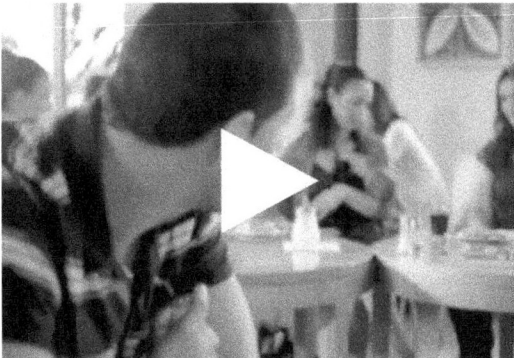

When You
Need a Feed

(Breastfeeding
Campaign from
New Zealand)

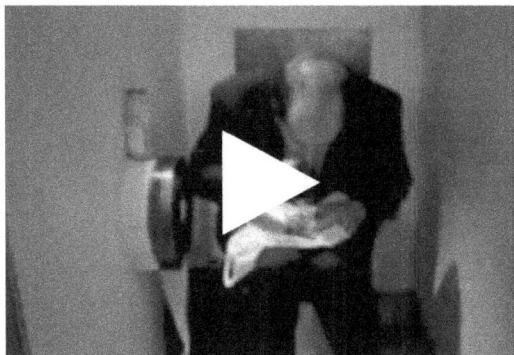

You Wouldn't
Eat Here

(from the Australian
Breastfeeding
Association)

Supporting Working Mothers

The U.S. Breastfeeding Committee's (USBC) Workplace Support in Federal Law Web page has been updated, including an expanded FAQ section, links to new federal resources, and this new report: *Better Health for Mothers and Children: Breastfeeding Accommodations under the Affordable Care Act*, from the Institute for Women's Policy Research: http://www.iwpr.org/publications/pubs/better-healthfor-mothers-and-children-breastfeeding-accommodations-under-the-affordable-care-act

The USBC page is here: http://www.usbreastfeeding.org/Workplace/WorkplaceSupport/ WorkplaceSupportinFederalLaw/tabid/175/Default.aspx

USLCA

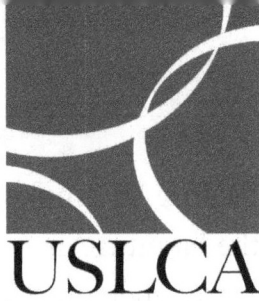

Working and Breastfeeding

Practical Ways You Can Support Employed Breastfeeding Mothers

Barbara D. Robertson, MA, IBCLC, RLC[1]

Keywords: breastfeeding, employment, *The Business Case for Breastfeeding*, pumping, working and breastfeeding, working mothers

The Business Case for Breastfeeding indicates that 80% of mothers stop breastfeeding within the first month of returning to work (Cardenas & Major, 2005). Unfortunately, research on returning to work and breastfeeding is limited. However, it is possible for clinicians to support working mothers and increase their rates of success. This article outlines some practical ways to support breastfeeding mothers as they return to work.

It is possible to support working mothers in reaching their breastfeeding goals. There are several critical factors for

---

1   barbara@bfcaa.com

supporting breastfeeding in employed mothers that I have identified in the literature and my clinical practice. Despite the dire statistics, mothers in my practice actually do well. None of them were quitting breastfeeding in the first month of returning to work. Providing accurate information about how breast milk supply works, and how to remove their breast milk, along with a little social and emotional support, seemed to help my clients keep breastfeeding, despite the occasional difficulty. I have identified five critical factors that help mothers meet their breastfeeding goals.

Breastfeeding Is Going Well Before Returning to Work

One critical factor for success is having the mother be good at breastfeeding before she returns to work. We know that breastfeeding becomes less work (and generally easier) for most mothers at about 6-7 weeks (Mohrbacher & Kendall-Tackett, 2010). If breastfeeding isn't going well, or a mother goes back to work before 6-7 weeks, she is more likely to be unsuccessful with this transition. If a mother is struggling with pain, has a baby who doesn't feed well at the breast, or her milk supply is low when she returns to work, she is doubly challenged from the get-go! Providing a plan to address these issues along with hope, accurate information, and support can help mothers continue breastfeeding, even as they return to work.

Support From an International Board Certified Lactation Consultant

The support and information that an International Board Certified Lactation Consultant (IBCLC) can provide are critical for a mother. Many mothers don't have anyone in their lives who understand or care about why they are even trying to continue to breastfeed and work. IBCLCs do care. We want her to be able to meet her breastfeeding goals. Together we can help shift those low statistics of working and breastfeeding success.

Success at Milk Removals

Another critical factor for success is how well the mother is removing her milk when separated from her baby. Most of my clients use a standard, personal use, double-electric breast pump. But as we know, not all pumps are created equal. Some work well, and some don't work as well. Using a brand of pump that has a good vacuum, different size breast shields (so important!), and variable speeds will increase her chance of success. At the same time, if a pump has all these things and she is still not getting out her breast milk, IBCLCs have to get creative. Maybe she needs to try a different brand of pump, rent a hospital-grade pump, use a hand pump, or hand express. Watching a mother pump is important. Test the vacuum. Make sure her shields fit well (Meier, 2004; Prime, Geddes, Spatz, Trengove, & Hartmann, 2010). Many mothers have no idea that different size breast shields even exist!

Positive Associations to Help Her "Feel the Love" for Her Pump

Make sure she is feeling the love for her pump. Without an oxytocin release, a mother is trying to pull the breast milk out of her body. With an oxytocin release, she is working in sync with her body. Her body is pushing the milk out of her breasts. This is much more effective. If she is having trouble "feeling the love," suggest warm compresses, warm breast shields (Kent, Geddes, Hepworth, & Hartmann, 2011), and/or massage before pumping (Bolman & Witt, 2013; Bowles, 2011). She can use "hands-on" pumping techniques to help get the breast milk flowing (Morton, n.d.). Also, hand expression for a minute or two on each breast after pumping can help with milk production (Morton et al., 2012).

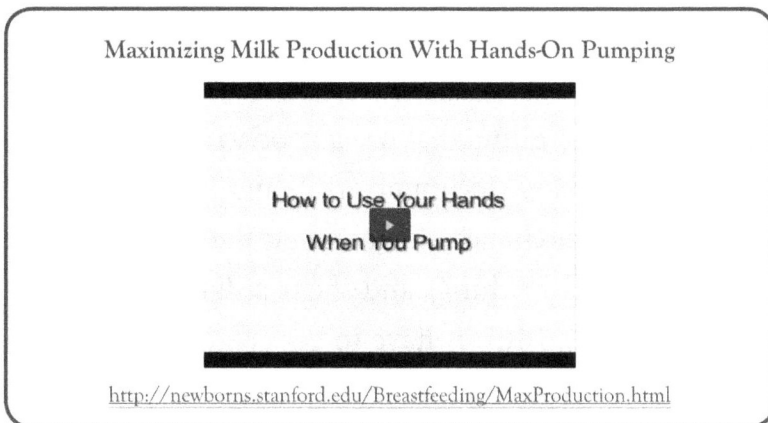

Maximizing Milk Production With Hands-On Pumping

How to Use Your Hands When You Pump

http://newborns.stanford.edu/Breastfeeding/MaxProduction.html

Some mothers find that visualizing their baby or their milk flowing helps. Others find that playing Candy Crush helps! There are some hypno-pumping visualization MP4 products out there (Freeze, 2014). Have them practice pumping while getting a massage, eating chocolate, or watching their favorite comedy. It's straight classical conditioning. Pair a condition with a response (think Pavlov's dog). Clients can help train their bodies to have an oxytocin surge in response to their pumps.

If a mother is having difficulties with her milk production, encourage her to blame her pump for lack of breast milk, not her body! If breast milk is not being removed effectively while she is separated from her baby, her supply will go down.

Know the Magic Number of Milk Removals

Mohrbacher (2012) proposes that each mother has a "magic number," which is the number of times that her milk must be removed in 24 hours to sustain her milk supply. A "milk removal" could be a breastfeed, a pumping session, or a hand expression session. When babies are being fed too much while away from mothers, they often only breastfeed from mom two or three times during a workday. Usually, this is once in the morning and once before bed. If mothers are pumping three times at work, two breastfeeds three pumps, it's five milk removals. Five milk removals in 24 hours are not very many. Some mothers can get away with this low number of milk removals, but most can't. Their breast milk supply starts to gradually decrease. By adding an extra pump before bed, I was helping the mother increase her milk removals and that seemed to help her supply. However, perhaps it would be easier if the baby needed to nurse four to six times on a workday. This would increase a mother's milk removals to seven to nine, which is more normal.

To help mothers keep track of all of this information in a fairly simple way, she will need to track just three numbers. I suggest that she total up how many ounces of breast milk she removes from her breasts in a week; how many ounces of breast milk the baby receives from the bottle in a week; and if she has a typical work week, how many times per 24 hours she moves her breast milk. I usually suggest tracking from midnight on Wednesday to midnight on Thursday.

1. How much milk did you pump or hand express per week?

2. How much breast milk did your baby consume while away from you per week?

3. How many times did you move your milk (a breastfeed, a pump, or a hand expression) from midnight Wednesday to midnight Thursday?

If clients track these numbers each week and any of these numbers start to shift, up or down, they can catch this quickly and get help. How many times have you worked with a mother and asked when she thinks this problem started and she answers, "Well, now that I am thinking about it, about 6 weeks ago?" So long ago! If she is counting weekly, she can catch changes right away. Let her know she should contact you immediately if she notices a negative change.

Supportive Child Care

Working and breastfeeding success can also be at risk if the mother's child care provider does not value her breast milk or her breastfeeding relationship with her baby. Overfeeding the baby while the mother is away is a common problem. The child care provider needs to understand that not all crying or fussiness is about food. They also need to know how to care for pumped breast milk, and how to bottle feed a baby in a breastfeeding-friendly manner by pacing the bottle feed (see Box 1). I actually recommend that all babies should be fed in this manner, not just breastfed babies or if there is breast milk in the bottle. Pacing the feed helps the baby control his or her intake and prevents overeating, which may help prevent obesity in later life.

Avoid Overfeeding at Childcare

The final stumbling block relates to overfeeding and subsequent diminished breastfeeding when moms and babies are reunited. When a baby has been overfed at childcare, not only is it almost impossible to keep providing enough pumped breast milk for the baby, but the baby also doesn't need to breastfeed as often from the mom when they get back together. It is as if the baby is saying, "No thanks; I'm good! I had all my needed calories for today from my caregiver." This does not hold true for all babies, but it does for many. Also, being away from mom can be stressful and tiring. Babies can sometimes sleep longer at night because of this. Between not needing to nurse because of the calorie overload during childcare and sleeping longer at night, mothers can end up breast-feeding far less than they were before returning to work. I have often suggested that moms pump before going to bed if their baby was going to sleep at 8:00 p.m. and not feed much during the night. This strategy appears to help improve their breast milk supply.

Box 1. "Pacing" the Bottle Feed

Pacing

- Helps babies feel safe and comfortable while they feed.
- Helps keep the flow more like breastfeeding.
- Helps reduce overfeeding of babies with a bottle.
- Helps protect the breastfeeding relationship.

How Pacing Works

- Have the baby sit very upright.
- Use a slow-flow, wide-base bottle teat.
- Touch the baby's chin or upper lip with the tip of the teat. When the baby cues for feeding by opening his or her mouth, gently slide the teat in as deeply as the baby allows.
- Keep the bottle so the breast milk just fills the teat. You want the baby to have to pull the milk out of the teat, not just pour into his or her mouth.
- Don't worry about the baby swallowing air. You may need to burp more but this is a small price to pay compared to training the baby to think that feeding is easy. You want to teach babies that feeding takes time and effort, with the breast and with the bottle.
- After three or so swallows, gently twist the teat so the nipple seal is broken and rest the teat against the baby's chin, cheek, or upper lip. This allows the baby to catch his or her breath and realize that feeding takes time but not worry that the breast milk and bottle are gone.
- Is the baby getting stressed? Is the baby frowning, wrinkling their forehead, widening their eyes, splaying their hands, making squeaking sounds, or choking? If so, gently twist the teat out of their mouth and give them a break.
- When the baby cues again by opening their mouth wide, repeat the process.
- This process should take about 20 minutes. The baby needs time to realize that they are full just like grown-ups. It takes a little more time but it is so worth it!
- Watch for satiation cues (e.g., getting sleepy, not cueing by opening the mouth, turning away from the teat, becoming more interested in the surroundings) and let them decide that they are done.
- If you feel that the baby has had an appropriate amount of supplement, take a break, have a burp, change a diaper, shift position, and see if the baby cues again. If so, offer another 0.5–1 ounce.

Not all babies can handle paced feeding, but most babies appreciate it.

Source: Kassing, D. (2002). Bottle-feeding as a tool to reinforce breastfeeding. Journal of Human Lactation, 18 (1), 56–60. Used with permission.

Summary

In my practice, I've found that five things can sabotage a mother's ability to continue breastfeeding after she returns to work: starting out with breastfeeding not working well, lack of information and support, milk removals not working well, lack of paced bottle feeding, and a mother's daily milk removals reducing over time are the most common culprits I have found in sabotaging a mother's success in meeting her breastfeeding goals when returning to work. Providing information about these issues may help a mother head off trouble before it starts, or at least help her quickly identify when she is moving down a slippery slope, and can greatly increase her odds of having the breastfeeding relationship she dreamed of before returning to work.

References

Bolman, M., & Witt, A. (2013). *The basics of breast massage and hand expression.* Retrieved from http://www.bfmedneo.com/BreastMassageVideo.aspx

Bowles, B. C. (2011). Breast massage: A "handy" multipurpose tool to promote breastfeeding success. *Clinical Lactation, 2*(4), 21–24. Retrieved from http://media.clinicallactation.org/2-4/ CL2-4bowles.pdf

Cardenas, R., & Major, D. (2005). Combining employment and breastfeeding: Utilizing a work-family conflict framework to understand obstacles and solutions. *Journal of Business and Psychology, 20*(1), 31–51.

Freeze, R. (2014). *Hypnosis for pumping breast milk and hypnosis for making more milk.* Retrieved from http://www.newbornconcepts.com/products.html

Kassing, D. (2002). Bottle-feeding as a tool to reinforce breastfeeding. *Journal of Human Lactation, 18*(1), 56–60.

Kent, J. C., Geddes, D. T., Hepworth, A. R., & Hartmann, P. E. (2011). Effect of warm breastshields on breast milk pumping. *Journal of Human Lactation, 27*(4), 331–338.

Meier, P. (2004). Choosing a correctly-fitted breastshield for milk expression. *Medela Messenger, 21*, 8–9.

Mohrbacher, N. (2012). The magic number and long-term milk production. *Clinical Lactation*, 2 (1), 15–18. Retrieved from http://www.clinicallactation.org/article.php?id=8&journal_id=5

Mohrbacher, N., & Kendall-Tackett, K. (2010). *Breastfeeding made simple: Seven natural laws for nursing mothers (2nd ed.).* Oakland, CA: New Harbinger Publications.

Morton, J. (n.d.). *Maximizing milk production with hands-on pumping.* Retrieved from http://newborns.stanford.edu/Breastfeeding/MaxProduction.html

Morton, J., Wong, R. J., Hall, J. Y., Lai, C. T., Lui, J., Hartmann, P. E., & Rhine, W. D. (2012). Combining hand techniques with electric pumping increases the caloric content of milk in mothers of preterm infants. *Journal of Perinatology*, 32 (10), 791–796. http://dx.doi.org/10.1038/jp.2011.195

Prime, D. K., Geddes, D. G., Spatz, D. L., Trengove, N. J., & Hartmann, P. E. (2010). The effect of breastshield size and anatomy on milk removal in women. *Journal of Human Lactation*, 26(4), 419–445.

Other Helpful References

Ahluwalia, I. B., Morrow, B., & Hsai, J. (2005). Why do women stop breastfeeding? Findings from the Pregnancy Risk Assessment and Monitoring System. *Pediatrics*, 116, 1408–1412.

Berggren, K. (2006). *Working without weaning.* Amarillo, TX: Hale Publishing.

Carothers, C., & Hare, I. (2010). The business case for breastfeeding. *Breastfeeding Medicine*, 5, 229–231.

Clark, A., Anderson, J., Adams, E., & Baker, S. (2008). Assessing the knowledge, attitudes, behaviors, and training needs related to infant feeding, specifically breastfeeding, of child care providers. *Maternal and Child Health Journal*, 12, 128–135.

Colburn-Smith, C., & Serrette, A. (2007). *The milk memos: How real moms learned to mix business with babies—And how you can, too.* New York, Penguin Books.

Fein, S. B., Mandal, B., & Roe, B. E. (2008). Success of strategies for combining employment and breastfeeding. *Pediatrics*, 122, S56–S62.

Walker, M. (2011). *Breastfeeding and employment: Making it work.* Amarillo, TX: Hale Publishing.

West, D., & Marasco, L. (2009). *Bottle nipples that minimize nipple confusion or flow preference.* Retrieved from http://www.lowmilksupply.org/nipples.shtml

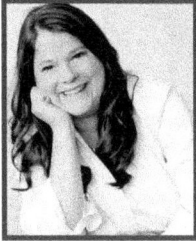

Barbara D. Robertson, MA, IBCLC, RLC, is the owner of The Breastfeeding Center of Ann Arbor and an associate editor of *Clinical Lactation.* Barbara was director of professional development for the U.S. Lactation Consultant Association from 2009 to 2014. She received the Michigan Breastfeeding Network Outstanding Community Breastfeeding Support Award in 2009.

USLCA

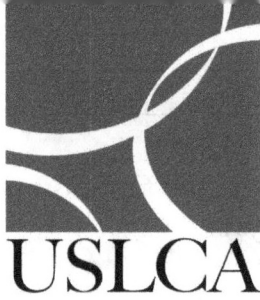

Use of World Health Organization and CDC Growth Charts for Children Aged 0-59 Months in the United States (Excerpt)

L.M. Grummer-Strawn, PhD,
C. Reinhold, PhD & N.F. Krebs, MD

Keywords: WHO growth charts, CDC growth charts, infant weight gain, lactation

In 2006, the Centers for Disease Control and Prevention (CDC), the National Institutes of Health, and the American Academy of Pediatrics convened an expert panel to review scientific evidence and discuss the potential use of the new WHO growth charts in clinical settings in the United States. On the basis of input from this expert panel, CDC recommends that clinicians in the United States use the 2006 WHO international growth charts, rather than the CDC growth charts, for children aged <24 months (available at https://www.cdc.gov/growthcharts). The CDC growth charts *should continue to be used for the assessment of growth in persons aged 2-19 years.*

Editor's Note: The following is an excerpt from an article prepared by L.M. Grummer-Strawn, C. Reinold, N.F. Krebs, and the Centers for Disease Control and Prevention.

Original reference: Grummer-Strawn, L.M., Reinold, C., & Krebs, N.F. (2010). Use of World Health Organization and CDC Growth Charts for children aged 0-59 months in the United States. Morbidity and Mortality Weekly Report, 59, September 10.

Introduction

The physical growth of infants and children has long been recognized as an important indicator of health and wellness (Cole, 2000; Garcia & de Onis, 2004). Growth charts have been used for at least a century to assess whether a child is receiving adequate nutrition and to screen for potentially inadequate growth that might be indicative of adverse health conditions. Traditionally, attention has focused on undernutrition. However, in the past few decades, concerns about excessive weight gain have increased, and growth charts have been used to screen for overweight, including obesity.

In April 2006, the World Health Organization (WHO) released a new international growth standard for children aged 0-59 months (WHO, 2006). Similar to the 2000 CDC growth reference (Kuczmarski et al., 2000; 2002), these growth charts describe weight for age, length (or stature) for age, weight for length (or stature), and body mass index (BMI) for age. WHO growth curves include BMI for age starting at birth, and CDC growth curves include BMI for age beginning at age 2 years. CDC and WHO growth charts also include a curve for head circumference for age; CDC provides values for children aged <36 months, and WHO charts include a head circumference curve for those aged <60 months.

Because two sets of growth curves exist for assessing child growth, clinicians in the United States need guidelines indicating which curves should be used and for which children. This report provides guidance on the use of the WHO and CDC growth charts, and is intended for health care providers and others who measure and assess child growth.

Creation of the WHO and CDC Growth Curves

Growth Reference Versus Growth Standard

The CDC and WHO growth charts differ in their overall conceptual approach to describing growth. The WHO charts are growth standards that describe how healthy children should grow under optimal environmental and health conditions. The curves were created based on data from selected communities worldwide, which were chosen according to specific inclusion and exclusion criteria. Deviation from the WHO growth standard should prompt clinicians to determine whether suboptimal environmental conditions exist, and if so, whether they can be corrected.

Whereas the WHO charts describe growth of healthy children in optimal conditions, the 2000 CDC growth charts are a growth reference, not a standard, and describe how certain children grew in a particular place and time. The CDC charts describe the growth of children in the United States during a span of approximately 30 years (1963–1994).

> The recommendation to use the 2006 WHO international growth charts for children aged <24 months is based on several considerations, including the recognition that breastfeeding is the recommended standard for infant feeding.

Rationale for Recommendations

Use of Growth Reference or Growth Standard in Clinical Settings

Opinions of the participants varied about whether the use of a growth standard or a growth reference would be best for clinical settings in the United States. Several participants explained that identification of growth that is unhealthy (i.e., indicates an underlying adverse health condition) or abnormal first requires a definition of healthy growth, thus a standard is needed. Other participants countered that because many children do not live in ideal environmental conditions, interpreting their growth by comparing them to a growth standard might not be appropriate. Likewise, some children who live in optimal conditions deviate from the normal growth curve but are not unhealthy. Participants acknowledged that adoption of a standard for assessing growth in children would create a substantial need for the education of clinicians, but would also create an opportunity for clinicians to identify and address environmental conditions that might be negatively affecting growth. Meeting participants agreed that in practice, clinicians often use growth references, such as the CDC growth charts, as a standard to evaluate healthy growth rather than a reference as intended.

Recommendations

Use of WHO Growth Charts for Children Aged <24 Months

Use of the 2006 WHO international growth standard for the assessment of growth among all children aged <24 months, regardless of type of feeding, is recommended (The charts are available at https://www.cdc.gov/growthcharts). When using the WHO growth charts, values of 2 standard deviations above and below the median, or the 2.3rd and 97.7th percentiles (labeled as the 2nd and 98th percentiles on the growth charts), 24 months is most feasible because measurements switch from recumbent length to standing height at this age, necessitating use of new printed charts.

Continued Use of CDC Growth Charts for Children Aged 24-59 Months

Use of the CDC growth charts for children aged 24-59 months is recommended. The CDC charts also should be used for older children because the charts extend up to age 20 years, whereas the WHO standards described in this report apply only to children aged 0-59 months. The rationale for continuing to use CDC growth charts includes the following: 1) the methods used to create the WHO and CDC charts are similar after age 24 months, 2) the CDC charts can be used continuously through age 19 years, and 3) transitioning at age 24 months is most feasible because measurements switch from recumbent length to standing height at the this age, necessitating use of new printed charts.

> When using the WHO growth charts to screen for possible abnormal or unhealthy growth, use of the 2.3rd and 97.7th percentiles (or ±2 standard deviations) are recommended, rather than the 5th and 95th percentiles.

Use of Recommended Growth Charts in Clinical Settings

CDC recommends the use of modified versions of the WHO curves for children aged <24 months that include the 2.3rd and 97.7th percentiles, and are appropriate for clinicians. These curves have been developed and are available at http://www.cdc.gov/growthcharts. Training tools for clinicians are being developed, and also will be available at this website.

Clinicians should recognize that the WHO charts are intended to reflect optimal growth of infants and children. Although many children in the United States have not experienced the optimal environmental, behavioral, or health conditions specified in the WHO study, the charts are intended for use with all children aged <24 months. Therefore, their growth might not always follow the patterns shown in the WHO curves. For example, formula-fed infants tend to gain weight more rapidly after approximately age 3 months and therefore cross upward in percentiles, perhaps becoming classified as overweight. Although no evidence-based guidelines for treating overweight in infancy exist, early recognition of a tendency toward obesity might appropriately trigger interventions to slow the rate of weight gain.

For the first 3 months of age, the WHO charts show a somewhat faster rate of weight gain than the CDC charts, leading to the identification of more infants who appear to be growing slowly. Clinicians should recognize that this slower rate of weight gain is typical for formula-fed infants. For breastfed infants identified as growing slowly, clinicians need to carefully assess general health issues and ensure appropriate management of lactation. Only if there is evidence of lactation inadequacy should they consider supplementation with formula.

Differences in the length-for-age WHO and CDC charts are small, and clinical differences based on these charts are expected to be insignificant. In contrast, when the WHO charts are used to assess the growth of

U.S. children, fewer children aged 6-23 months will be identified as having inadequate weight for age. Some assert that this might be beneficial because overdiagnosis of underweight might damage the parent-child interaction, subjecting families to unnecessary interventions and possibly unintentionally creating an eating disorder (Wright et al., 1994). However, children who are identified as having low weight for age on the WHO charts will be more likely to have a substantial deficiency. Clinicians need to seek out the causes for poor growth and propose changes accordingly. For example, poor weight gain might result from neglect, substantial morbidities, or other medical problems that require immediate attention.

> Clinicians should be aware that fewer U.S. children will be identified as underweight using the WHO charts, slower growth among breastfed infants during ages 3–18 months is normal, and gaining weight more rapidly than is indicated on the WHO charts might signal early signs of overweight.

References

Cole, T.J. (2003). The secular trend in human physical growth: A biological view. *Economics & Human Biology, 1*, 161–168.

Garza, C., & de Onis, M. (2004). Rationale for developing a new international growth reference. *Food & Nutrition Bulletin, 25*(Suppl 1), S5–12.

Kuczmarski, R.J., Ogden, C.L., Grummer-Strawn, L.M., et al. (2000). CDC growth charts: United States. *Advance Data, 314*, 1–27.

Kuczmarski, R.J., Ogden, C.L., Guo, S.S., et al. (2002). 2000 CDC growth charts for the United States: Methods and development. *Vital Health Statistics, 246,* 1–190.

World Health Organization. (2006). *WHO child growth standards: length/height-for-age, weight-for-age, weight-for-height and body mass index-for-age: Methods and development.* Geneva, Switzerland: World Health Organization; 2006. Available at http://www.who. int/childgrowth/publications/technical_report_pub/en/index. html. Accessed June 1, 2010.

Wright, J.A., Ashenburg, C.A., & Whitaker, R.C. (1994). Comparison of methods to categorize undernutrition in children. *Journal of Pediatrics, 124,* 944–946.

24-Hour Cribside Assistance. A Manual for New Dads.

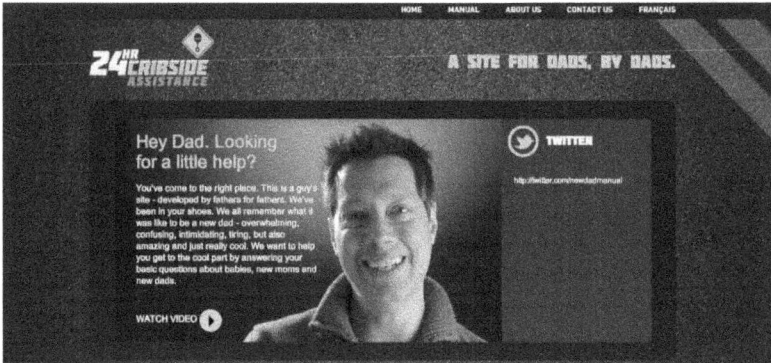

http://www.newdadmanual.ca/

USLCA

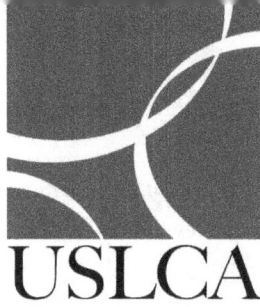

Can Lactation Consultants Find Appropriate Uses for the World Health Organization Growth Curves?

Susan E. Burger, MHS, PhD, IBCLC, RLC[1]

Sara D. Newman, JD, CLC, PCD (DONA[2])

Keywords: breastfeeding, growth monitoring, growth charts, growth curves, growth standards, World Health Organization, lactation consultants

The release of the World Health Organization growth curves in 2006 enabled lactation consultants and other health care practitioners to compare the growth of infants and young children against normal, healthy breastfed infants for the first time. Prior to that, lactation consultants only had access to reference curves that included the less-healthy growth

1   Lactescence, NYC, sburgernutr@nyc.rr.com
2   D is for Doula, New York City

patterns of formula-fed infants. Systematic reviews suggest that while growth curves are widely used, the impact of their use on children's health and nutrition remains unclear. Program experience has shown growth curves may be useful for promotion of other health services and for education and motivation, but may not be as useful for screening at-risk infants. In light of this experience, lactation consultants might find the best use of growth curves would be to educate mothers, families and other health care practitioners about the healthier growth patterns of breastfed infants, and to promote feeding practices accordingly.

Evolution of Growth Curves

Growth curves have evolved from many different references to a single standard (See Diagram 1)[3]. Part of this progression was triggered by the realization that when infants and young children are raised under optimal conditions of nutritional intake and health, ethnicity has a negligible influence on their growth (Habicht et al., 1974). So while there is no need for population-specific curves, how infants are fed does matter. Technical committees convened by the WHO reached the conclusion that the healthy breastfed infant should be the standard against which all other infants are compared (Garza & de Onis, 2004). In 2010, the United States Centers for Disease Control and Prevention (CDC) adopted this standard (GrummerStrawn et al., 2010), and the International Board of Lactation Consultant

---

3   The article, "Use of World Health Organization and CDC Growth Charts for children aged 0-59 months in the United States," mentioned in this volume provides a succinct summary of the history of growth curves. http://www.cdc.gov/mmwr/preview/mmwrhtml/rr5909a1.htm?s_cid=445909al_e

Examiners included it in the clinical competencies for lactation consultants (IBCLE, 2010).

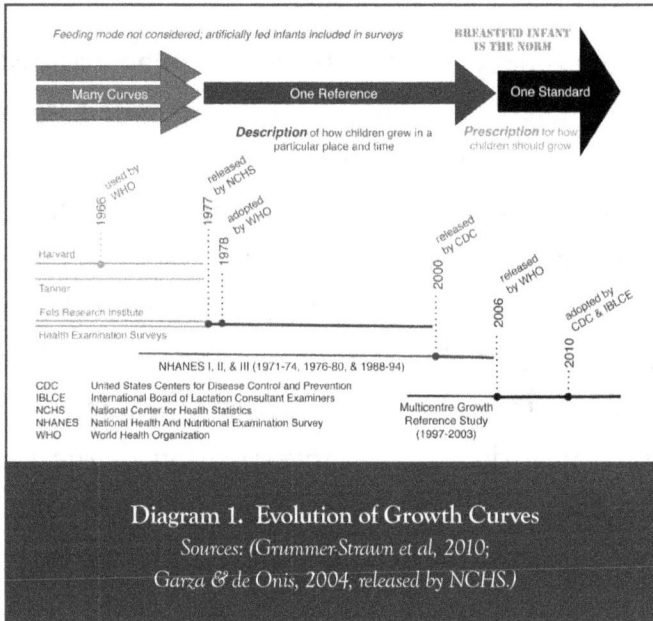

Diagram 1. Evolution of Growth Curves
Sources: (Grummer-Strawn et al, 2010;
Garza & de Onis, 2004, released by NCHS.)

Prior Use of Growth Curves

In the 1970s, David Morley pioneered the concept of monitoring growth plotted against a reference curve as a "Road to Health" (Morley, 1973). In the 1980s, James P. Grant, Executive Director of the United Nations Children's Fund (UNICEF), propelled this concept into greater international prominence by advocating for growth promotion as one of four key low-cost interventions considered likely to reduce childhood death (Rohde, 2010). Growth monitoring is neither an intervention, nor even a diagnostic tool; it is merely a screening tool to identify growth patterns that may not be healthy. The process of monitoring growth is only likely to be useful if the underlying causes of any deviations are determined and appropriate actions are taken to promote healthy growth.

The authors of an investigation into how Ministries of Health use growth monitoring concluded, "growth monitoring is an intrinsic part of pediatric care around the world" (de Onis et al., 2004). Out of the 178 of the Ministries of Health whose representatives responded to the questionnaire, 154 (86%) sent hard copies of growth charts, and 165 (93%) reported taking actions in response to growth faltering. Reported actions included hospital referrals, nutrition advice, investigation of the causes, closer follow-up, direct medical care, and home visits. The authors admitted they could not ascertain the extent to which those actions actually took place, nor the impact of growth monitoring on child nutrition.

The authors of a systematic review of weight monitoring in developed and developing countries found no reliable evidence to support or refute the opinion that "investment into the activity has worthwhile benefits, and does no harm" (Garner et al., 2000). Only two studies, both in developing countries, met the author's scientific criteria for assessing the impact of growth monitoring (Panpanich & Garner, 1999).

Children's growth improved in 12 villages in Tamil Nadu, India that received nutrition and health education from a village nutrition worker. There did not, however, appear to be any additional improvement in the six villages that were randomly assigned to use growth curves along with the education (George et al., 1993).

In nine primary health care centers in Lesotho, mothers participated in a program that provided growth monitoring, individual counseling, and group nutrition education about complementary feeding and diarrheal management. Mothers who were instructed in the use of growth charts[4] understood the meaning of the charts better than the mothers who received no instruction (Ruel et al., 1990). Mothers understood the concepts of weight gain and loss better than stagnant weight. Most of the significant improvement in knowledge about specific targeted messages on complementary feeding and feeding during diarrhea appeared to be due to growth monitoring, education, and counseling (Ruel & Habicht, 1992). Education in the use of growth charts appeared to only have a marginally significant impact on the knowledge about diarrheal management among mothers with less than secondary school education, new clinic attendants and mothers of malnourished children. Of note, it was the at-risk mothers of malnourished children whose understanding that breastfeeding should be continued during diarrhea who appeared to benefit from the additional education in the use of the WHO charts.

The author of another review looked more deeply into the purpose and process of how growth monitoring and

---

4   This study compared two types of growth charts, one based on the percent of a standard represented as a linear band and another based upon percentile curves.

promotion was being conducted (Ruel, 1995). This review concluded that growth monitoring has the potential to be "extremely useful in Primary Health Care programs, particularly for education, motivation, and to promote other health services" (p. 93). The improvements included an increased frequency of home visits and checkups, and increased coverage of vaccines, micronutrient supplements, and oral rehydration. Success depended upon the "active involvement of mothers, families, and communities in all stages of the design, implementation and evaluation" (p. 93).

Growth charts may be less useful for screening. Under usual field conditions, rates of misclassifying children were high, at around 25% (Ruel, 1995). Sources of misclassification included random measurement errors, systematic errors from scales that were not calibrated, errors when rounding off digits, and errors in age determination. Inaccurate plotting was the second most frequent problem reported by Ministry of Health representatives (de Onis et al., 2004).

The evidence collected on the use of growth curves has focused on growth faltering. Yet, the CDC recognizes that concerns about excessive weight gain have increased in the last several decades, and growth curves have been used to screen for overweight and obesity (Grummer-Strawn et al., 2010). While the WHO curves are better designed to identify overweight and obese children than older references (WHO, 2008c), the CDC feels more research is needed to guide how to use this information effectively for this purpose (Grummer-Strawn et al., 2010).

Existing Training Modules for the WHO Curves

The WHO developed the downloadable Training Course on Child Growth Assessment for health care providers who measure and assess the growth of children or who supervise these activities (WHO, 2008a). The general information in the easy-to-read modules and related job aids for how to measure, plot, interpret, and counsel mothers using the growth curves provides useful pragmatic tips that can be useful reminders, even for experienced lactation consultants. Although the manual is geared for developing areas, it could be easily adapted for practitioners working in developed areas. Only one of the four case studies in the counseling module (WHO, 2008b) is relevant for lactation consultants. Unfortunately, one aspect of that case seems physiologically unlikely and the corresponding recommendation seems more likely to diminish the supply than to improve growth.

The CDC is developing a training module for the use of the WHO curves (Grummer-Strawn et al., 2010). If lactation consultants are involved in the development of this module, they might add more depth and relevance for suggested actions to improve breastfeeding.

Potential Use of Growth Curves by Lactation Consultants

Empirical evidence is not yet available on whether the use of the WHO growth curves by IBCLCs will benefit or harm breastfeeding practices, nor have any specific tools been developed for them. Prior experience suggests the WHO growth curves may not be useful as a screening tool due to misclassification errors. Furthermore, using deviations from the growth curves to predict risk might be akin to using malnutrition rates to predict famine. By the time malnutrition rates have increased, it is too late; children have already suffered the consequences of the famine. Therefore, lactation consultants should not expect the curves to replace other assessments and history taking, particularly those that may prevent unhealthy changes in growth from occurring in the first place.

Since many lactation consultants work in hospitals, and rarely assess infants beyond the early initiation of breastfeeding, the International Lactation Consultant Association (ILCA) guidelines for the expected weight loss and regain of birth weight (ILCA, 2005) are likely to be more appropriate for this early period than plotting curves. A controlled trial in Scotland suggests that weighing frequently enough to track weight loss and regain of birth weight does not discourage breastfeeding when it is coupled with targeted breastfeeding support (McKie et al., 2006). Plotting the weights would only make sense if it provided some additional information for making decisions. In fact, the interval of the first two weeks is so compressed on the CDC version of the WHO curves that the dots for weights cluster so compactly, that they are almost unreadable.

Once babies are past the first two weeks, it becomes possible to start plotting an upward curve of growth.

The conclusions of the authors of a small ethnography study of the use of growth monitoring by health visitors during clinics and breastfeeding groups in Northern England (Sachs et al., 2006), reads like a "What Not to Do" manual for this stage of infancy. Infants were weighed more frequently than recommended. Mothers wanted their infants to gain along a percentile curve, preferably the 50th. Mothers appeared to be concerned about even minor fluctuations in weight gain of no likely biological consequence. The focus by health workers and mothers on weight gain, rather than breastfeeding effectiveness, led them to intervene with formula, early introduction of solids, and changes in maternal diet. The lack of a comparison group leaves open the possibility that it was not the curves, per se, but the advice that was the problem.

Lactation consultants are far more likely to provide advice that leads to improvements in breastfeeding practices than other health care practitioners. Furthermore, lactation consultants have in-depth insights into feeding practices that may lead to overfeeding and contribute to the rising rates of childhood obesity.

Yet weighing, recording, and plotting curves is time intensive and may detract from collecting other more pertinent information and counseling mothers. The finding that growth curves appeared to improve the understanding of at-risk mothers hints that selective use might be appropriate for specific, targeted purposes. This approach might exploit the educational, motivational, and promotional potential of this tool, while maintaining the primary focus on improving breastfeeding practices.

Anecdotal Observations of Selective Use of Growth Curves in a Breastfeeding Clinic

Over the course of the last 12 months, growth monitoring was initiated on a selective basis in a drop-in group clinic in Manhattan (Burger, 2010-2011).[5] The criterion for plotting curves was that maternal anxiety about maintaining or improving practices was not alleviated by other forms of information. A few examples included the following.

» Weight gain appeared slow along the NCHS curves, but normal or less slow along the WHO curves.

» Sleep training reduced the frequency of breastfeeds to the point that weight gain dropped substantially along the WHO curves.

» Weight gain continued to be normal along the WHO curves when supplements were withdrawn after improvements in breastfeeding practices.

Gathering the information and plotting the curves was time consuming and had to be conducted outside the clinic. The visual illustration of growth complemented other counseling techniques used to assist these women to gain confidence in their ability to feed their infants and recognize their cues. Several of the curves illustrated to mothers how misclassification along the CDC curves led

---

5   The problems encountered in the Manhattan drop-in clinic are likely to reflect the specific clientele that attend this clinic. Lactation consultants working with different populations in different settings are likely to see different problems.

to inappropriate assumptions about the infant's growth and recommendations for feeding practices.

Case Study: Illustration of Fluctuations in Weight and Length Gain.[6]

The mother and baby were initially seen at home on day 7 and attended drop-in and semi-private clinics. The curves were plotted using data from the WHO expanded tables for constructing national health cards (WHO, no date) for weight-for-age (Graph 1), length-for-age (Graph 2), and weight-for-length (Graph 3). The baby's weight and length were plotted using the measurements taken by the baby's pediatrician. Measurements were converted to kilograms and centimeters using standard conversions.

At the first visit, the mother was recuperating from complications from labor and delivery and experiencing severe nipple pain. The baby had been supplemented with formula in the hospital in response to a diagnosis of jaundice. The mother continued to visit a drop-in and semi-private group clinic. With a combination of pumping and improved positioning she was able to eliminate the use of formula by week 4. The baby was able to feed exclusively from the breast by week 9.

The mother felt breastfeeding was going relatively well and her baby was very content and active until he was 4 months old and started to teethe. He became fretful

---

6   Permission was obtained from the mother to present growth curves and relevant information about her infant that contributed to changes in growth.

and unsettled while he was teething. Shortly thereafter, the mother and baby also traveled to visit her family for several weeks. When they returned home, she felt that she and her baby were out of sync and out of sorts due to the change in time zones and teething. She experienced a bout of mastitis when her baby was around 5 months old. Four teeth fully erupted by the time the baby was 6 months old.

The mother reported that she felt the pediatrician was extremely concerned about the slowing in weight compared to the CDC references curve during the interval between 4 and 6 months. The slowing in weight gain over this interval is apparent, but not as dramatic, when compared to the WHO standards (Graph 1). The baby's weight in relation to his length dropped around the time he started teething (fourth dot on Graph 3). The length gain only slowed down once the baby started teething (Graph 2). Prior to 4 months, the baby's gain in length initially was more rapid than the WHO standard and then steady along a standard curve, even while the weight gain was slightly slower than the standard.

Minimizing Misinterpretation

If lactation consultants do choose to use the WHO curves, it is important to minimize the misclassification that may lead to incorrect interpretations and inappropriate interventions. Measurement errors are common and can increase misclassification.

Graph 1. Weight-for-age compared to WHO standards.

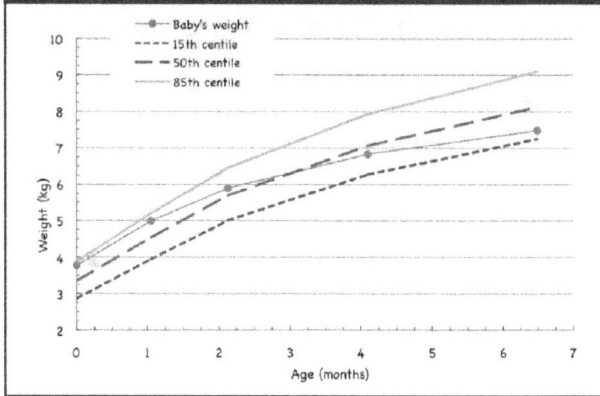

Graph 2. Length-for-age compared to WHO standards.

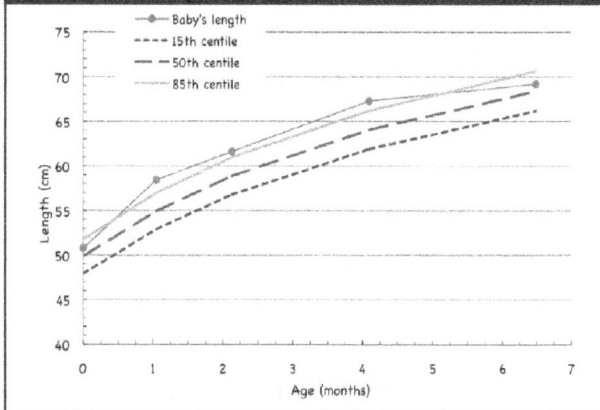

Graph 3. Weight-for-length compared to WHO standards.

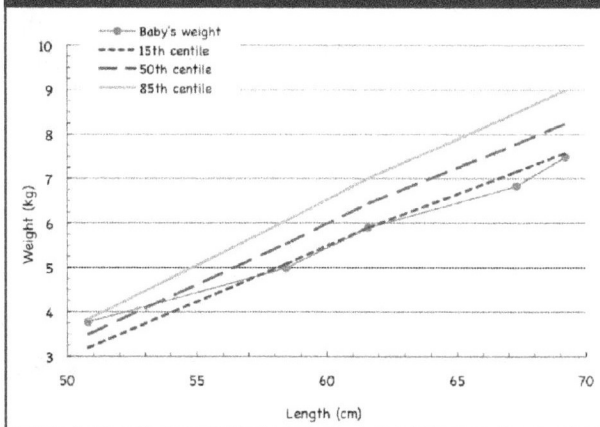

Simple common-sense steps should be routinely implemented to minimize error when weighing infants.

Additional steps can minimize misclassification when determining the baby's age at the time of measurement (Diagram 3).

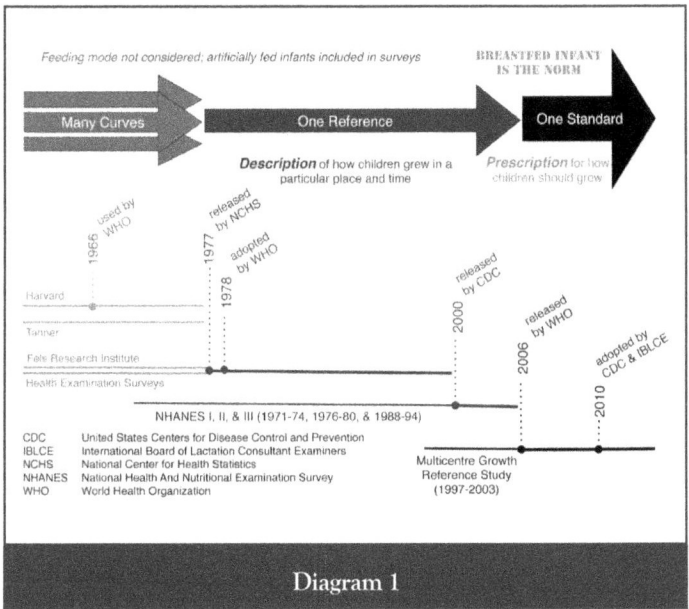

Diagram 1

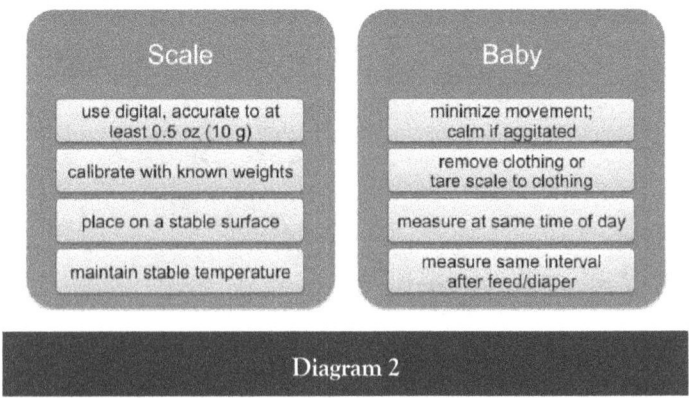

Diagram 2

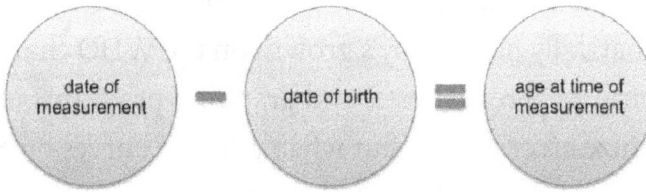

Diagram 3

When it comes to the indicators of growth, the vast majority of countries use weight-for-age (97%); more than half as the sole indicator (de Onis et al., 2004). Less than half reported using length/height-for-age (41%), and less than one third (23%) use weight-for-length/height. Yet measuring length is necessary for a differential diagnosis of stunting (low length-for-age), underweight (low weight-for-length), and obesity (high weight-for-length). If weight gain is abnormal, lactation consultants should consider measuring or assessing already recorded length as well. Length should also be measured in ways that minimize errors (Diagram 4).

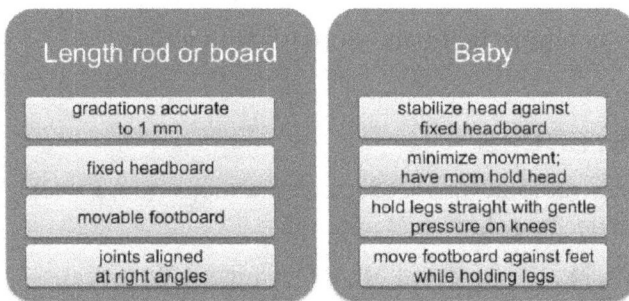

Length rod or board	Baby
gradations accurate to 1 mm	stabilize head against fixed headboard
fixed headboard	minimize movment; have mom hold head
movable footboard	hold legs straight with gentle pressure on knees
joints aligned at right angles	move footboard against feet while holding legs

Diagram 4

Prepackaged computer programs, applications that automatically plot a baby's growth on the WHO charts, or customized spreadsheets, and graphing programs might minimize errors that occur when plotting curves by hand.

Conclusions

While there are theoretical benefits and potential harms of using growth curves, there is insufficient evidence to draw any firm conclusions. Past experience suggests that growth curves may not as useful as a screening tool as they might be for educational, motivational, and promotional purposes. Routine use of growth monitoring in breast-feeding clinics and groups is likely to be time consuming and detract from time spent on proven assessment and counseling methods. Lactation consultants might be in the best position to explore selective use of the new WHO growth curves to motivate, promote, and educate mothers and other health care practitioners about the healthy growth of the breastfed infant, and practices that will foster breastfeeding. Such targeted use would need to be specifically tailored to the varied populations and settings where lactation consultants work.

References

Burger, S. (2010-2011). Anecdotal observations from a weekly dropin breastfeeding clinic in Manhattan.

de Onis, M., Winjhoven, T.M., & Onyango, A.W. (2004). Worldwide practices in child growth monitoring. *Journal of Pediatrics, 144*, 461-465. http://www.jpeds.com/article/S00223476%2804%2900017-4/abstract

de Onis, M., Garza, C., Onyango, A.W., & Borghi E. (2007). Comparison of the WHO Child growth standards and the CDC 2000 growth charts. *Journal of Nutrition, 137*, 144-148. http://jn.nutrition.org/content/137/1/144.abstract?sid=528b3ed9-cff84ced-8a9b-9ea74295049f

Garner, P., Panpanich, R., & Logan S. (2000). Is routine growth monitoring effective? A systematic review of trials. *Archives of Disease in Childhood, 82*, 197-201. http://adc.bmj.com/ content/82/3/197.abstract?sid=0aacc64c-8d26-43d2-9c81ee2ab4a552ae

Garza, C., & de Onis, M. (2004). Rationale for developing a new international growth reference. *Food and Nutrition Bulletin. 25*(1), Supplement 1, S5-S13. http://www.who.int/childgrowth/mgrs/fnu/en/index.html

George, S.M., Latham, M.C., Abel, R., Ethirajan, N., & Frongillo, E.A. Jr. (1993). Evaluation of effectiveness of good growth monitoring in south Indian villages, *Lancet, 342*, 348-352. http://www.thelancet.com/search/results?searchTerm=George%2C%20 S&fieldName=AllFields&op=and&searchterm2=&fieldname2= AllFields&year=1993&volume=342&page=348&jrnl=lan&artyp es=&advsrch=t&journalFromWhichSearchStarted=&sort=date& order=desc&collectionName=Medline

Grummer-Strawn, L.M., Reinold, C., & Krebs, N.F. (2010). Use of World Health Organization and CDC growth charts for children aged 0-59 months in the United States. *Morbidity and Mortality Weekly Report, 59*, RR-9. http://www.cdc.gov/mmwr/preview/ mmwrhtml/rr5909a1.htm?s_cid=445909al_e

Habicht J.-P., Martorell, R., Yarbrough, C., Malina, R.M., & Klein, R.E. (1974). Height and weight standards for preschool children: How relevant are ethnic differences in growth potential? *Lancet, 1*, 611-614.

International Lactation Consultant Association (ILCA). (2005). *Clinical guidelines for the establishment of exclusive breastfeeding*, p 6. http://www.ilca.org/files/resources/ClinicalGuidelines2005.pdf

International Board of Lactation Consultant Examiners (IBCLE). (Updated December 6, 2010). *Clinical competencies for the practice of International Board Certified Lactation Consultants.* http://www. iblce.org/professional-standards

McKie, A., Young, D., & Macdonald, P.D. (2006). Does monitoring newborn weight discourage breastfeeding? *Archives of Diseases in Childhood, 91*, 44-46. http://adc.bmj.com/content/91/1/44. abstract?sid=d8840b2b-83e3-4c4a-8368-a611931df21f

Morley, D. (1973). *Paediatric priorities in the developing world.* London: Butterworth.

Panpanich, R., & Garner, P. (1999). Growth monitoring in children. *Cochrane Database of Systematic Reviews, 4*, Art No.: CD001443. http://www2.cochrane.org/reviews/en/ab001443.html

Rohde, J.E. (2010). *"The James P. Grant lecture: an unfinished agenda for children." Keynote address.* http://fieldnotes. unicefusa.org/2010/04/jim_grant_and_the_unfinished_a.html

Ruel, M.T., Pelletier, D.L., Habicht, J.-P., Mason, J.B., Chobokoane, C.S., & Maruping, A.P. (1990). Comparison of mothers' understanding of two growth charts in Lesotho. Bulletin of the *World Health Organization, 68*, 483-491. http://whqlibdoc.who.int/bulletin/1990/Vol68-No4/

Ruel, M.T., & Habicht, J-P. (1992). Growth charts only marginally improved maternal learning from nutrition education and growth monitoring in Lesotho. *The Journal of Nutrition, 122*, 1772-1780 http://jn.nutrition.org/content/122/9/1772.full.pdf+html

Ruel, M. (1995). Growth monitoring as an educational tool. In P. Pinstrup-Andersen, D. Pelletier & H. Alderman (Eds.), *Child growth and nutrition in developing countries: Priorities for action* (pp. 78-96). Ithaca, NY: Cornell University Press.

Sachs, M., Fiona, D., & Carter, B. (2006). Feeding by numbers: An ethnographic study of how breastfeeding women understand their babies' weight charts. *International Breastfeeding Journal, 1*, 29. http://www.internationalbreastfeedingjournal.com/ content/1/1/29

World Health Organization (WHO). (2006). *WHO Multicentre Growth Reference Study Group. WHO Child Growth Standards: Length/height-for-age, weight-for-age, weight-for-length, weight-for-height and body mass index-for-age: Methods and development.* http://www. who.int/childgrowth/standards/technical_report/en/index.html

World Health Organization (WHO). (2008a). *Training course on Child Growth Assessments: WHO Child Growth Standards.* http://www. who.int/childgrowth/training/en/

World Health Organization (WHO). (2008b). D: *Counselling on growth and feeding. Training course on Child Growth Assessments: WHO Child Growth Standards.* http:// www.who.int/childgrowth/standards/wfa_boys_p_exp.txt

World Health Organization (WHO). (2008c). *A: Introduction. Training course on Child Growth Assessments: WHO Child Growth Standards.* http://www.who.int/childgrowth/standards/lhfa_boys_p_exp.txt

World Health Organization (WHO). (no date). *Expanded tables for constructing national health cards. Child growth standards.* http://www.who.int/childgrowth/standards/wfl_boys_p_exp.txt

USLCA

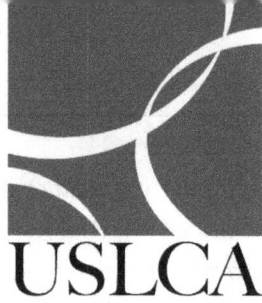

Overcoming Breastfeeding Challenges:
A Qualitative Inquiry

Debra Rose Wilson, PhD, MS, RN, IBCLC, RLC, AHN-BC CHT[1]
Cathy Cooper, EdD, MSN, RN, CNE[2]
Kristi Plunk, MSN, RN[3]
Mariesa Severson, MSN, RN, WHNP[4]

Keywords: challenges, breastfeeding, resilience, duration, early weaning, qualitative, Parse

Breastfeeding duration rates continue to fall short of recommended targets. Weaning that is earlier than the mother intended likely occurs when she encounters a challenge that she could not overcome. It is not clear from existing studies why some women overcome challenges while others do not. This qualitative phenomenological study asked, "What is the lived experience of overcoming breastfeeding challenges?" Three themes emerged through grounded-theory

1   Debrarosewilson@comcast.net, Middle Tennessee State University, Walden University
2   Cathy.cooper@mtsu.edu, Middle Tennessee State University
3   Kristina.Plunk@mtsu.edu, Middle Tennessee State University
4   Mariesa.Severson@mtsu.edu, Middle Tennessee State University

data analysis. Anticipatory Guidance instilled hope and knowledge, and identified potential resources, all of which assisted with overcoming the challenges. Breastfeeding is complexly interwoven with Maternal-Role Attainment. Resilience provides protective factors when one is challenged. Theory arising from these themes has implications for both practitioners and researchers. This study illustrates concrete strategies to enhance maternal-role attainment and ensure desired duration of breastfeeding.

Breastfeeding is a proactive and cost-effective way of reducing global rates of child mortality and morbidity. More mothers in North America are choosing to breastfeed. Initiation rates are increasing but duration rates are not increasing as rapidly as hoped. The purpose of this qualitative study was to examine and describe the lived experience of women who initiated breastfeeding, overcame challenges in the process, and continued to breastfeed successfully. Application of the theory developed from these findings may provide avenues to increase the ability of mothers to overcome breastfeeding challenges.

The Centers for Disease Control and Prevention (2012) report that 81.9% of U.S. mothers initiated breastfeeding, with 60.6% still breastfeeding at 6 months. Approximately 46.2% of babies are exclusively breastfed through three months, and 25.5% are exclusively breastfed through 6 months. Health Canada (2012) reports that 87.9% of mothers initiate breastfeeding and rates are steadily rising. National and global initiatives have contributed to a steady increase in these indicators over the past five years. Breastfeeding-friendly hospitals, workplaces, and communities have developed programs to educate and facilitate breastfeeding. However, many hospitals have policies that do not conform to the WHO code and may interfere with a mother's success (CDC, 2012). To compound this, duration rates are lower than desired and likely even lower than reported (Agampodi et al., 2011; Chalmers et al., 2009).

Most health authorities recommend breastfeeding exclusively for up to 6 months, with continued breast-feeding for 2 years or longer. Women often discontinue breastfeeding before intended, but there are other mothers who face these same challenges, overcome them, and continue to breastfeed (Li et al., 2008). While it seems obvious that mothers with previous breastfeeding experience should breastfeed longer, studies have found parity does not influence the overall duration of breast-feeding (Ladomenou et al., 2007).

The duration of breastfeeding is influenced by education and age of the mother, prenatal intent, race, and social support (Pollard & Guill, 2009). Factors that influence the decision to discontinue breastfeeding include availability of formula, perception of inadequate supply, prematurity, lack of social support, cultural acceptance, and return to work (Pollard & Guill, 2009). The existing literature, however, does not clearly identify what intrinsic or extrinsic factors differentiate the mother who gives up breastfeeding when challenged from the mother who overcomes the same challenge and continues to successfully breastfeed. By understanding the process and factors contributing to success, health care providers can better predict challenges, identify mechanisms to motivate and support the mother, and decrease the rate of early weaning.

This study was guided by phenomenology, existentialism, and Parse's theory of Human Becoming. Phenomenological theory is driven by the belief that the subjective life experience is the relevant definition of personal reality. Phenomenology describes the structure of the subjective experience as presented to consciousness (Husserl, 1965). Existentialist enquiry tends to focus on the characteristics of ontology, or modes of being (Sartre, 1993). The phenomenological approach is congruent with the practice of lactation consulting because of the holistic focus on the human experience (Parse, 1998). Parse's mid-range nursing theory of Human Becoming emphasizes perception and meaning from the patient's perspective, and recognizes the patient's responsibility for making informed choices (Parse, 1997, 1998). Meaning arises from the exchange of the human with all that is surrounding, and defines life.

Method

A qualitative phenomenological design was used to examine the lived experience of overcoming breastfeeding challenges. IRB approval and informed consent were obtained. Seventeen mothers who overcame breastfeeding challenges were interviewed and audiotaped. Interviews were open-ended, lasted from 45 to 65 minutes, and were conducted by the same IBCLC researcher trained in qualitative interviewing and true presence.

The participant was encouraged to tell the story of her breastfeeding experience, the challenges she faced, the strategies used to overcome challenges, the personal qualities employed, the transcendence through the experience, and the resultant meaning found in the experience. Verbatim transcripts were analyzed using grounded theory, an inductive approach to explore patterns and generate theory. After data analysis and model development, two independent practitioners took the model to mothers who overcame breastfeeding challenges and verified the model as valid and reflective of their experience.

Findings

Demographic data collected from the 17 participants reflected an age range of 20 to 34 years, with a mean of 28 years. Sixty-five percent (11) of the participants were primipara, and 35% (6) were multipara. Annual household income ranged from less than $15,000 to $150,000–$249,000, with a median of approximately $52,000. The mean age of the baby at the time of the interview was 12 months, with a minimum of 5 months and a maximum of 23 months. The majority of the participants 13 (76%) were Caucasian, 2 (18%) were Hispanic, and 2 (18%) were African American. Seven participants (41%) had completed some college, 6 (35%) were high school graduates, 3 (18%) had Bachelor's degrees, and 1 (1%) had completed some high school.

Three themes emerged from the categories and codes generated by the data. These themes included: 1) Anticipatory guidance; 2) Breastfeeding as complexly intertwined with maternal-role attainment; and 3) Resilience. The theory generated from this study describes how the anticipation and perception of success in breastfeeding influences the experience and is reflective of learned and innate resilience to overcoming breastfeeding challenges.

THEME 1: Anticipatory Guidance

Participants, whether primaparas or multiparas, drew upon guidance, resources, and teaching they had obtained prior to delivery. Most mothers had sought out education through formal means, such as breastfeeding classes, or through less-formal means, such as the internet, friends and family, and reading books on the subject.

> *My confidence might be higher than other women who didn't go to breastfeeding classes. I just expected to be able to do this, 'cause that's what I learned in the classes. I can do this; I will make enough milk for my baby. A mom who doesn't have that confidence might give up easier.*

Regardless of the source of prenatal education and support, mothers reported a connection they had made that gave them confidence, which encouraged their expectation and resolve to overcome the challenge. Mothers reported being more tenacious with problem solving, and actively seeking out more problem solving approaches when previous strategies had failed.

When I still had troubles latching the baby after all the help already, I still just KNEW that I could do this. I kept digging into the resources, finding new ones, then finally finding a Lactation Consultant who could break it down for me and teach me the movements. My aunt kept telling me this was why she had given up breastfeeding, and it was OK if he [the baby] needed a bottle. It wasn't like I was her. I was like a dog with a bone, and I wasn't giving up.

The mother's expectation of success played a part in overcoming challenges. Support systems were in place prior to delivery, which allowed more efficient access to help. The participants valued advice from nurses, family, and friends who had successfully breastfed. They reported actively seeking help early when problems arose.

I was not going to tolerate these really sore nipples for very long. I knew it wasn't supposed to hurt so bad. I called [sister] and she got me to call for help right away.

Anticipatory guidance was first introduced in mental health education in the early 1930s. Using anticipatory guidance as a primary intervention, health care providers can alleviate stress and apprehension. Support, skill development, and informational needs are met by providing preemptive information so that role mastery can occur (Hill et al., 1994). A prenatal education program that includes one-to-one education, behavioral and skill development counseling, and breastfeeding classes, is the single most effective primary intervention to increase initiation and duration of breastfeeding (Keister et al., 2008). When partners and family of the childbearing women were included in the education, it further increased the mothers' sense of support and confidence.

THEME 2: Breastfeeding Is Complexly Intertwined with Maternal-Role Attainment

Kitzinger (1987) first described the experience of breast-feeding in a holistic framework to provide anticipatory guidance for the lactating mother.

> *Mechanical failure and difficulties with breastfeeding at the physiological level cannot be isolated from the psychological aspects of lactation, and psychology is interlocked with social factors ... (p. 198).*

The embodied experience of breastfeeding was seen as fundamental to the definition of motherhood.

> *If I couldn't feed my baby, what was I doing trying to have a baby? ... not just as a failure at breastfeeding, but that meant I sucked as a mother too. I know that's extreme, but that's how you hear it when you are all upset.*

Mercer introduced the concept of maternal-role development in the early 1960s. Later, Rubin introduced it in middle-range theory (Tarkka, 2003). Maternal-role development is primarily a cognitive process, highly interacting with social aspects of culture and family that influences development as a mother. Feedback from people in women's support networks validates their competence, and mothers' success is influenced by the expectations of others (Tarkka, 2003). A statement that breastfeeding will be successful, and setting an expectation for overcoming any challenges, should be common practice for those educating, assisting, or supporting the childbearing family.

My heart just sunk when I was encouraged to quit breast-feeding by well-meaning family ... This [breastfeeding] was something that only I could do for my baby, and I didn't want that taken away from me ... I wanted that special connection, that made me feel like I was the only one who could care for my baby ... this was my baby and this was what I was supposed to do.

THEME 3: Resilience

Resilience, the third theme identified from the data, is characterized by positive adaptation and is:

... the capacity to rebound from adversity, strengthened and more resourceful. It is an active process of endurance, self-righting, and growth in response to crisis and challenge (Walsh, 2006, p. 4).

In general, resilience is defined in terms of a person's capacity to adapt and/or persevere despite difficult circumstances. This perseverance is a capacity to withstand stressors without psychological dysfunction. Resilience is built and improved upon with the development of new coping skills. It is a dynamic quality, closely related to hardiness, resourcefulness, self-efficacy, and self-confidence. Resilient individuals possess a particular set of attitudes, as well as the cognitive and emotional skills necessary to adapt, survive (and perhaps even thrive) in the midst of hardship or adversity. Resilient individuals view challenges as opportunities, manage a variety of situations competently, possess faith with deeply rooted meaning, and have a healthy support network. Resilience enables people to find the determination to meet and overcome challenges in the midst of overwhelming events. Strategies for developing or improving resilience include developing positive and strong relationships with friends and family, identifying a purpose for one's life, building on the skills and strategies from previous experiences that were successful in overcoming difficulties, and engaging in self-care activities, such as regular exercise, adequate sleep, and eating a healthy diet (Mayo Clinic Staff, 2009).

A strong sense of coherence and resilience enhances existing coping skills, acts as a buffer to adversity, and contributes to an understanding that challenges are to be expected. Previous studies have demonstrated a significant relationship between self-efficacy and breastfeeding success (Pollard & Guill, 2009). Pollard and Guill (2009) identified self-efficacy as a modifiable factor to reduce early weaning. Women with a higher perceived self-efficacy tended to persist, even through challenges. Women with lower self-efficacy or self-confidence may wean earlier than they intended. Some will avoid challenges if they feel they do not have the skills to cope. While Pollard and Guill's study is a great beginning to examining modifiable risk factors, self-efficacy is only one of numerous factors that contribute to resilience.

> Even though it took a while to get through that, and I wanted to quit, I knew I had what it took; to keep trying.

There may be some predictive value to screening for self-efficacy and resilience. At-risk populations would benefit from intentional targeting of education and support. In the resilience literature, there has been little attention devoted to ethnically diverse populations and socioeconomic differences. There were no specific differences noted between populations in this qualitative study, but the role of racial socialization in the development of resilience has been well established (Terzian & Harriott, 2010). Health care providers would benefit from a culturally diverse perspective when assessing or fostering resilience behaviors.

The concept of resilience was previously studied only within the domain of psychology. There is a trend towards more multidisciplinary use of resilience as a research construct, although there were no published studies found that examined resilience as a factor in breastfeeding. Focus on enhancing resilience, as a characteristic malleable to support, education, and anticipatory guidance, is within the realm of practice for lactation consultants, nurses, midwives, and childbirth educators.

Generated Theory

Figure 1 illustrates the concepts and themes associated with overcoming breastfeeding challenges. Anticipatory guidance was a significant factor in generating hope, building a knowledge base, and lining up potential resources for support. Successful attainment of the maternal role is complexly integrated into successful breastfeeding; the belief that breastfeeding defined good mothering provided more motivation to overcome challenges. Resilience was a protective factor also fed by hope, knowledge, and resources.

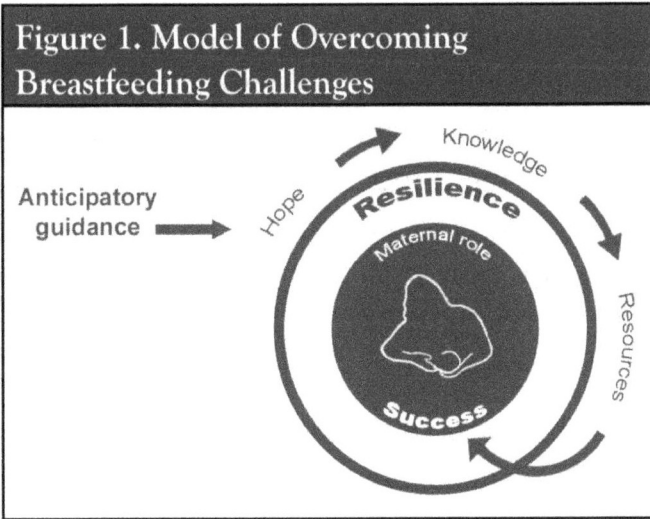

Figure 1. Model of Overcoming Breastfeeding Challenges

Limitations

Generalization about the meaning of breastfeeding cannot be derived from a small sample. This study was intended to suggest likely avenues of inquiry for further research. Exploring the meaning of overcoming challenges and successfully breastfeeding opens up the door to other paradigms of thought.

Recommendations

Further research is needed to test the theory derived from the current data. Quantitative data should be gathered on personality types, resilience, instillation of hope, and other objectively measured characteristics to determine which of these factors are relevant to overcoming breastfeeding challenges. Expanded studies could compare the charac-teristics of those who weaned by choice to those mothers who weaned before personal goals were met. New data may further validate meaning and theory that emerged when exploring the lived experience of successful breastfeeding. It is clear that anticipatory guidance about breastfeeding improves outcomes. Inexpensive educational strategies during prenatal care, as well as a pre-conception normalization of successful breastfeeding, will have an impact on increasing duration of breastfeeding.

Unintentional weaning often happens within the first weeks postpartum. During this critical period, developing support systems would help increase the duration of breastfeeding. Identification of those mothers who may be at risk for stopping breastfeeding early would help steer program funds to appropriate recipients. Early maternal reemployment has been associated with increased weaning (Ladomenou et al., 2007). Systems of support in the workplace to promote breastfeeding should be acknowledged and rewarded by professional and parenting groups.

Not only is patient education important, but education and support of health care providers is warranted. Continued support, education, and resources will add to successful breastfeeding and have an impact on achieving *Healthy People 2020* targets of longer breastfeeding duration.

Conclusions

Readers are not going to be surprised that mothers who overcame breastfeeding challenges reported being well prepared and organized with anticipatory guidance. Resources were in place if needed, and support systems were readily accessed. Breastfeeding is a holistic, lived experience, one that participants perceived as integral to the experience of motherhood. A health professional's approach to assisting breastfeeding mothers needs to be accurate, evidence-based, and holistic in approach. Anticipatory guidance prenatally and in the immediate postpartum period should provide information about common lactation problems, suggestion of strategies and resources to overcome these problems, and instillation of hope with an expectation of successful breastfeeding. Similar to previous work, these results support the value of identifying predicting factors for early weaning, and providing anticipatory guidance, knowledge, resources, and hope. This study describes the lived experiences of 17 mothers who successfully overcame challenges to breastfeeding. May their stories serve as a powerful example of resilience, a reminder to offer anticipatory education, and a source of encouragement for other women persevering through difficulties.

References

Agampodi, S. B., Fernando, S., Dharmaratne, S. D., & Agampodi1, T. C. (2011). Duration of exclusive breastfeeding: Validity of retrospective assessment at nine months of age. *BMC Pediatrics*, 11(80), 1-5. Retrieved from: http://www.biomedcentral. com/1471-2431/11/80

Centers for Disease Control and Prevention [CDC]. (2011). Vital signs: Hospital practices to support breastfeeding—United States, 2007 and 2009. *Morbidity and Mortality Weekly Report*, 60(30), 1020-1025.

Centers for Disease Control and Prevention [CDC]. (2012). *Breastfeeding Report Card—United States, 2011.* Retrieved from: http://www.cdc.gov/breastfeeding/data/reportcard.htm

Chalmers, B., Levitt, C., Heaman, M., O'Brien, B., Sauve, R., Kaczorowski, J., Maternity Experiences Study Group of the Canadian Perinatal Surveillance System, & Public Health Agency of Canada. (2009). Breastfeeding rates and hospital breastfeeding practices in Canada: A national survey of women. *Birth, 36*(2), 122-132.

Health Canada. (2012). *Breastfeeding data.* Retrieved from: http://www.hc-sc.gc.ca/index-eng.php

Hill, P., Humenick, S., & West, B. (1994). Concerns of breastfeeding mothers: The first six weeks postpartum. *Journal of Perinatal Education, 3*(4), 47-58.

Husserl, E. (1963). *Phenomenology and the crisis of philosophy.* (Q. Lauer, Trans.) New York: Harper and Row.

Keister, D., Roberts, K. T., & Werner, S. L. (2008). Strategies for breastfeeding success. *American Family Physician, 78*(2), 225-232.

Kitzinger, S. (1987). *The experience of breastfeeding.* New York: Penguin.

Ladomenou, F., Kafatos, A., & Galanakis, E., (2007). Risk factors related to intention to breastfeed, early weaning, and suboptimal duration of breastfeeding. *Acta Paediatrica, 96*(10), 1441-1444. doi: 10.1111/j.1651-2227.2007.00472.x

Li, R., Fein, S. B. Chen, J., & Grummer-Strawn, L. M. (2008). Why mothers stop breastfeeding: Mothers' self-reported reasons for stopping during the first year. *Pediatrics, 122*(Supplement 2), S69 -S76. doi: 10.1542/peds.2008-1315i

Mayo Clinic Staff. (2009). *Resilience: Build skills to endure hardship.* Retrieved from: http://mayoclinic.com/health/ resilience/ MH00078

Parse, R. R. (1997). *The human becoming school of thought: A perspective for nurses and other health professionals.* Thousand Oaks, CA: Sage Publications.

Pollard, D & Guill, M. (2009). The relationship between baseline self-efficacy and breastfeeding duration. *Southern Online Journal of Nursing Research, 9*(4). Retrieved from: http://www.

resourcenter.net/images/SNRS/Files/SOJNR_articles2/
Vol09Num04Art09.pdf

Sartre, J. P. (1993). *Being and nothingness: A phenomenological essay on ontology.* (H. W. Barnes, Trans.) New York: Washington Square Press. (Original work published in 1943).

Tarkka, M. (2003). Predictors of maternal competence by first-time mothers when the child is 8 months old. *Journal of Advanced Nursing, 4*(3), 233-240.

Terzian, M., & Harriott, V. (2010). From racial discrimination to substance use: The buffering effects of racial socialization. *Child Development Perspectives, 4*(2), 131-137.

Walsh, F. (2006). *Strengthening family resilience.* New York: The Guilford Press.

Dr. Debra Rose Wilson has a PhD in Health Psychology, with a focus in psychoneuroimmunology, and a MSN in holistic nursing

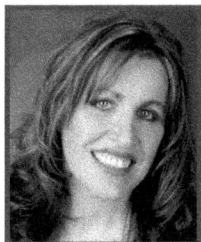

with a focus on CAM. Debra is a professor in the School of Nursing at Middle Tennessee State University and Walden University, and was an L&D and NICU nurse, and a prenatal educator. She is currently conducting research on stress and immune function, and maintains a private practice in lactation and hypnosis, and is working on another graduate degree in physics.

Dr. Cathy Cooper is an Associate Professor of Nursing at Middle Tennessee State University in Murfreesboro, TN, where she teaches Medical-Surgical Nursing. Her research interests include teaching and learning of adults, women and heart disease, and self-efficacy.

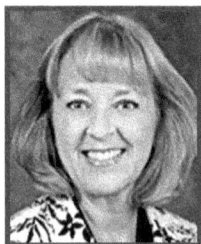

Kristi Plunk is a graduate of Lowenberg School of Nursing at the University of

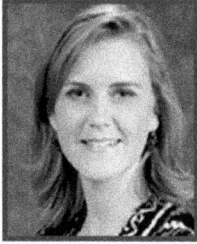

Memphis in Memphis, TN. She earned her BSN and MSN from University of Memphis. Kristi has 11 years' experience as a Labor & Delivery nurse, and is currently a clinical professor for Middle Tennessee State University in Murfreesboro, TN.

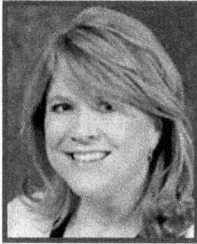

Mariesa Severson earned her MSN and BSN degrees at Arizona State University. She has been a nurse for over 25 years, specializing in Women's Health and Obstetrics, and serving as an L&D, postpartum, and neonatal nurse, as well as a women's health nurse practitioner and nurse educator. She is currently an ICEA, certified childbirth educator and a full-time assistant professor at Middle Tennessee State University in Murfreesboro, TN.

USLCA

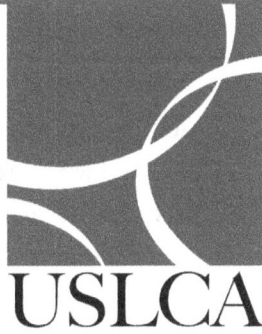

USLCA is a non-profit membership association focused on advancing the International Board Certified Lactation Consultant (IBCLC) in the United States through leadership, advocacy, professional development, and research.

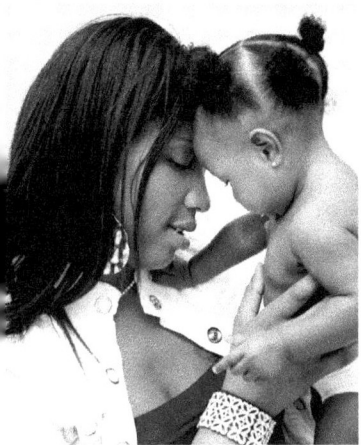

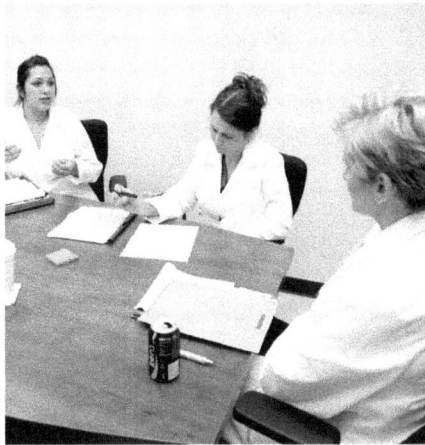

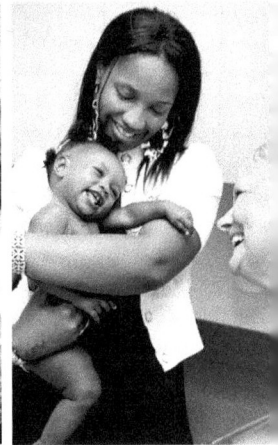

The U.S. Lactation Consultant Association Presents

Clinical Lactation Monographs

Professional Development

Milk Supply

Breast and Nipple Pain

Cultural Competence

Intrapartum Care

Lactation Management II

Lactation Management I

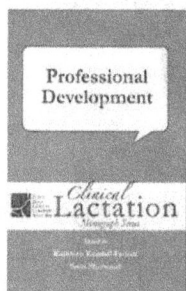

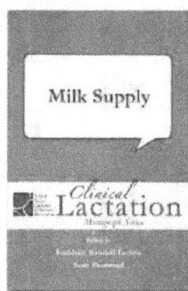

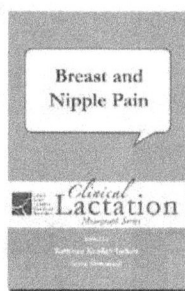

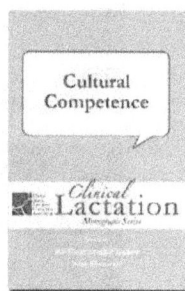

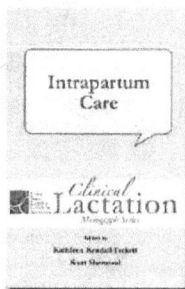

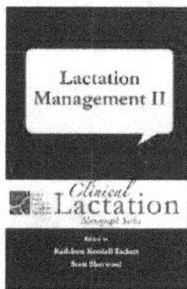

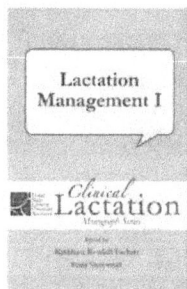

Praeclarus Press
Excellence in Women's Health

www.PraeclarusPress.com

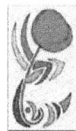

Breastfeeding and Women's Health Titles from Praeclarus Press

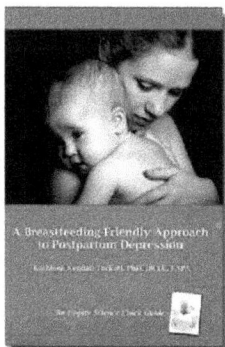

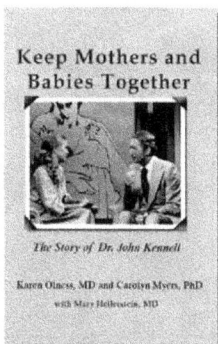

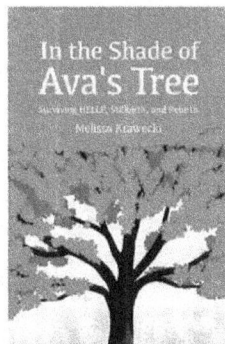

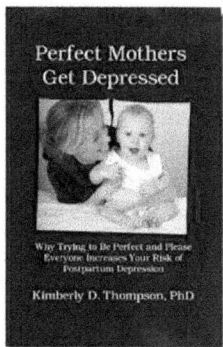

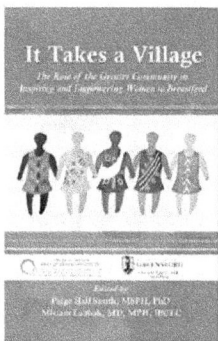

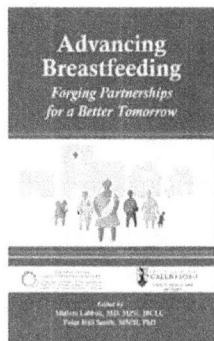

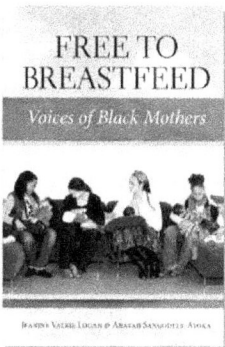

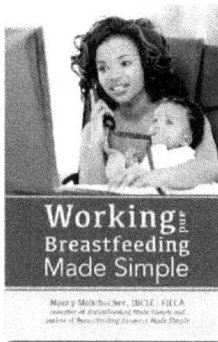

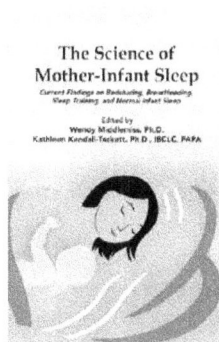

A Breastfeeding Friendly Approach to Postpartum Depression

Kathleen Kendall-Tackett, PhD, IBCLC, FAPA

The Praeclarus Science-Based Guide

Keep Mothers and Babies Together

The Story of Dr. John Kennell

Karen Olness, MD and Carolyn Myers, PhD
with Mary Helfenstein, MD

In the Shade of Ava's Tree

Surviving HELLP, Stillbirth, and Preterm Birth

Melissa Krawecki

Perfect Mothers Get Depressed

Why Trying to Be Perfect and Please Everyone Increases Your Risk of Postpartum Depression

Kimberly D. Thompson, PhD

It Takes a Village

The Role of the Greater Community in Inspiring and Empowering Women to Breastfeed

Edited by
Paige Hall Smith, MSPH, PhD
Miriam Labbok, MD, MPH, IBCLC

Advancing Breastfeeding

Forging Partnerships for a Better Tomorrow

Edited by
Miriam Labbok, MD, MPH, IBCLC
Paige Hall Smith, MSPH, PhD

FREE TO BREASTFEED

Voices of Black Mothers

JEANINE VALRIE LOGAN & AMAYAH SANGODELE-AYOKA

Working & Breastfeeding Made Simple

Nancy Mohrbacher, IBCLC, FILCA
coauthor of *Breastfeeding Made Simple* and author of *Breastfeeding Answers Made Simple*

The Science of Mother-Infant Sleep

Current Findings on Bedsharing, Breastfeeding, Sleep Training, and Normal Infant Sleep

Edited by
Wendy Middlemiss, Ph.D.
Kathleen Kendall-Tackett, Ph.D., IBCLC, FAPA

Praeclarus Press
Excellence in Women's Health

www.PraeclarusPress.com

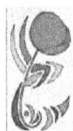

www.ingramcontent.com/pod-product-compliance
Lightning Source LLC
Chambersburg PA
CBHW070859280326
41934CB00008B/1507